FIRST AID FOR THE® PSYCHIATRY CLERKSHIP

FIFTH EDITION

LATHA GANTI, MD, MS, MBA, FACEP, FAHA
Vice Chair for Research and Academic Affairs
HCA UCF Emergency Medicine Residency
Program of Greater Orlando
Associate Medical Director, Polk County Fire Rescue
Professor of Emergency Medicine and Neurology
University of Central Florida College of Medicine
Orlando, Florida

SEAN M. BLITZSTEIN, MD
Staff Psychiatrist
Jesse Brown VA Medical Center
Director, Psychiatry Clerkship
Clinical Associate Professor of Psychiatry
University of Illinois at Chicago
Chicago, Illinois

MATTHEW S. KAUFMAN, MD
Medical Director
Emergency Department
Jersey City Medical Center
Bayonne, New Jersey

New York / Chicago / San Francisco / Athens / London / Madrid / Mexico City
Milan / New Delhi / Singapore / Sydney / Toronto

First Aid for the® Psychiatry Clerkship, Fifth Edition

Copyright © 2019 by McGraw-Hill Education. All rights reserved. Printed in the United States of America. Except as permitted under the United States Copyright Act of 1976, no part of this publication may be reproduced or distributed in any form or by any means, or stored in a data base or retrieval system, without the prior written permission of the publisher.

Previous editions copyright © 2016 by McGraw-Hill Education and copyright © 2011, 2005, 2002 by The McGraw-Hill Companies, Inc.

First Aid for the® is a registered trademark of McGraw-Hill Education. All rights reserved.

1 2 3 4 5 6 7 8 9   LOV   23 22 21 20 19 18

ISBN 978-1-260-14339-3
MHID 1-260-14339-2

Notice

Medicine is an ever-changing science. As new research and clinical experience broaden our knowledge, changes in treatment and drug therapy are required. The authors and the publisher of this work have checked with sources believed to be reliable in their efforts to provide information that is complete and generally in accord with the standards accepted at the time of publication. However, in view of the possibility of human error or changes in medical sciences, neither the authors nor the publisher nor any other party who has been involved in the preparation or publication of this work warrants that the information contained herein is in every respect accurate or complete, and they disclaim all responsibility for any errors or omissions or for the results obtained from use of the information contained in this work. Readers are encouraged to confirm the information contained herein with other sources. For example and in particular, readers are advised to check the product information sheet included in the package of each drug they plan to administer to be certain that the information contained in this work is accurate and that changes have not been made in the recommended dose or in the contraindications for administration. This recommendation is of particular importance in connection with new or infrequently used drugs.

This book was set in Warnock-Light by MPS Limited.
The editors were Bob Boehringer and Rhiannon Wong.
The production supervisor was Catherine Saggese.
Project management was provided by Ruma Khurana, MPS Limited.

This book is printed on acid-free paper.

Cataloging-in-publication data for this book is on file at the Library of Congress.

International Edition ISBN 978-1-260-56611-6; MHID 1-260-56611-0. Copyright © 2019 by McGraw-Hill Education. Exclusive rights by McGraw-Hill Education for manufacture and export. This book cannot be re-exported from the country to which it is consigned by McGraw-Hill Education. The International Edition is not available in North America.

McGraw-Hill Education books are available at special quantity discounts to use as premiums and sales promotions, or for use in corporate training programs. To contact a representative please visit the Contact Us pages at www.mhprofessional.com.

CONTENTS

Contributing Authors   v

Introduction   vii

Chapter 1: How to Succeed in the Psychiatry Clerkship   1

Chapter 2: Examination and Diagnosis   11

Chapter 3: Psychotic Disorders   21

Chapter 4: Mood Disorders   35

Chapter 5: Anxiety, Obsessive-Compulsive, Trauma, and Stressor-Related Disorders   49

Chapter 6: Personality Disorders   63

Chapter 7: Substance-Related and Addictive Disorders   79

Chapter 8: Neurocognitive Disorders   97

Chapter 9: Geriatric Psychiatry   111

Chapter 10: Psychiatric Disorders in Children   119

Chapter 11: Dissociative Disorders   133

Chapter 12: Somatic Symptom and Factitious Disorders   139

Chapter 13: Impulse Control Disorders   147

Chapter 14: Eating Disorders   153

Chapter 15: Sleep-Wake Disorders   161

Chapter 16: Sexual Dysfunctions and Paraphilic Disorders   173

Chapter 17: Psychotherapies   181

Chapter 18: Psychopharmacology   191

Chapter 19: Forensic Psychiatry   211

Index   219

CONTRIBUTING AUTHORS

SEAN M. BLITZSTEIN, MD
Staff Psychiatrist
Jesse Brown VA Medical Center
Director, Psychiatry Clerkship
Clinical Associate Professor of Psychiatry
University of Illinois at Chicago
Chicago, Illinois
Personality Disorders
Sexual Dysfunctions and Paraphilic Disorders

AMBER C. MAY, MD
Chief Fellow, Child and Adolescent Psychiatry Fellowship
University of Illinois at Chicago
Chicago, Illinois
Anxiety, Obsessive-Compulsive, Trauma and Stressor-Related Disorders
Neurocognitive Disorders
Psychiatric Disorders in Children
Dissociative Disorders

KELLEY A. VOLPE, MD
Assistant Professor of Clinical Psychiatry
Director, Child and Adolescent Psychiatry Fellowship
Medical Director, Pediatric Stress and Anxiety Disorders Clinic
University of Illinois at Chicago
Chicago, Illinois
Eating Disorders
Sleep-Wake Disorders
Psychotherapies
Forensic Psychiatry

BRANDI M. JACKSON, MD
Chief Resident, Department of Psychiatry
University of Illinois at Chicago
Chicago, Illinois
Examination and Diagnosis
Mood Disorders
Geriatric Psychiatry
Psychopharmacology

SURYA SABHAPATHY, MD
Chief Resident, Department of Psychiatry
University of Illinois at Chicago
Chicago, Illinois
Psychotic Disorders
Substance-Related and Addictive Disorders
Somatic Symptom and Factitious Disorders
Impulse Control Disorders

INTRODUCTION

This clinical study aid was designed in the tradition of the First Aid series of books. It is formatted in the same way as the other books in this series. However, a stronger clinical emphasis was placed on its content in relation to psychiatry. You will find that rather than simply preparing you for success on the clerkship exam, this resource will help guide you in the clinical diagnosis and treatment of many problems seen by psychiatrists.

Each of the chapters in this book contains the major topics central to the practice of psychiatry and has been specifically designed for the medical student learning level, to excel in the clerkship (shelf exams), as well as the USMLE Step 2 and 3 exams.

The content of the text is organized in the format similar to other texts in the First Aid series. Topics are listed by bold headings, and the "meat" of the topics provides essential information. The outside margins contain mnemonics, diagrams, exam and ward tips, summary or warning statements, and other memory aids. Exam tips are marked by the ♀ icon, tips for the wards by the ✋ icon, and clinical scenarios by the 🚶 icon.

CHAPTER 1

HOW TO SUCCEED IN THE PSYCHIATRY CLERKSHIP

Why Spend Time on Psychiatry?	2
How to Behave on the Wards	2
Respect the Patients	2
Respect the Field of Psychiatry	2
Take Responsibility for Your Patients	2
Respect Patients' Rights	3
Volunteer	3
Be a Team Player	3
Keep Patient Information Handy	3
Present Patient Information in an Organized Manner	3
How to Prepare for the Clerkship (Shelf) Exam	4
Study with Friends	4
Study in a Bright Room	4
Eat Light, Balanced Meals	4
Utilize Question Banks and/or Take Practice Exams	4
Pocket Cards	5

Your psychiatry clerkship will undoubtedly be very interesting and exciting. A key to doing well in this clerkship is finding the balance between drawing a firm boundary of professionalism with your patients while maintaining a relationship of trust and empathy.

Why Spend Time on Psychiatry?

For most, your medical school psychiatry clerkship will encompass the entirety of your formal training in psychiatry during your career in medicine.

Being aware of and understanding the features of mental dysfunction in psychiatric patients will serve you well in recognizing psychiatric symptoms in your patients, regardless of your specialty choice.

While anxiety and depression can worsen the prognosis of patients' other medical conditions, medical illnesses can cause significant psychological stress, often uncovering a previously subclinical psychiatric condition. The stress of extended hospitalizations can strain normal mental and emotional functioning beyond their adaptive reserve, resulting in transient psychiatric symptoms.

Psychotropic medications are frequently prescribed in the general population. Many of these drugs have significant medical side effects and drug interactions. You will become familiar with these during your clerkship and will encounter them in clinical practice regardless of your field of medicine.

Because of the unique opportunity to spend a great deal of time interacting with your patients, the psychiatry clerkship is an excellent time to practice your interview skills and "bedside manner."

How to Behave on the Wards

RESPECT THE PATIENTS

Always maintain professionalism and show the patients respect. Be respectful when discussing cases with your residents and attendings.

RESPECT THE FIELD OF PSYCHIATRY

- Regardless of your interest in psychiatry, take the rotation seriously.
- You may not agree with all the decisions that your residents and attendings make, but it is important for everyone to be on the same page.
- Dress in a professional, conservative manner.
- Because of the intense emotional suffering experienced by psychiatric patients, working with them can be overwhelming. Keep yourself healthy.
- Psychiatry is a multidisciplinary field. It would behoove you to continuously communicate with nurses, social workers, and psychologists.
- Address patients formally unless otherwise told.

TAKE RESPONSIBILITY FOR YOUR PATIENTS

Know as much as possible about your patients: their history, psychiatric and medical problems, test results, treatment plan, and prognosis. Keep your intern or resident informed of new developments that they might not be aware of, and ask them for any updates you might not be aware of. Assist the team in developing a plan; speak to consultants and family members. Never deliver bad news to patients or family members without the assistance of your supervising resident or attending.

RESPECT PATIENTS' RIGHTS

1. All patients have the right to have their personal medical information kept private. This means do not discuss the patient's information with family members without that patient's consent, and do not discuss any patient in public areas (e.g., hallways, elevators, cafeterias).
2. All patients have the right to refuse treatment. This means they can refuse treatment by a specific individual (the medical student) or of a specific type (electroconvulsive therapy). Patients can even refuse lifesaving treatment. The only exceptions to this rule are if the patient is deemed to not have the capacity to make decisions or if the patient is suicidal or homicidal.
3. All patients should be informed of the right to seek advance directives on admission. Often, this is done by the admissions staff or by a social worker. If your patient is chronically ill or has a life-threatening illness, address the subject of advance directives with the assistance of your resident or attending.

VOLUNTEER

Be enthusiastic and self-motivated. Volunteer to help with a procedure or a difficult task. Volunteer to give a 20-minute talk on a topic of your choice, to take additional patients, and to stay late.

BE A TEAM PLAYER

Help other medical students with their tasks; teach them information you have learned. Support your supervising intern or resident whenever possible. Never steal the spotlight or make a fellow medical student look bad. If your work for the day is completed, offer to help with tasks on other patients on your team, even if they are not your primary patients; helping to get work done may free up time for the resident or attending to spend more time teaching.

KEEP PATIENT INFORMATION HANDY

Use a clipboard, notebook, or index cards to keep patient information, including a history and physical, lab, and test results, at hand. However, make sure to keep all confidential patient information secure.

PRESENT PATIENT INFORMATION IN AN ORGANIZED MANNER

Here is a template for the "bullet" presentation:

> "This is a [**age**]-year-old [**gender**] with a history of [**major history such as bipolar disorder**] who presented on [**date**] with [**major symptoms, such as auditory hallucinations**] and was found to have [**working diagnosis**]. [**Tests done**] showed [**results**]. Yesterday, the patient [**state important changes, new plan, new tests, new medications**]."

This morning the patient feels [**state the patient's words**], and the mental status and physical exams are significant for [**state major findings**]. Plan is [**state plan**]."

The newly admitted patient generally deserves a longer presentation following the complete history and physical format.

Many patients have extensive histories. The complete history should be present in the admission note, but during ward presentations, the entire history is often too much to absorb. In these cases, it will be very important that you generate a **good summary** that is concise but maintains an accurate picture of the patient.

How to Prepare for the Clerkship (Shelf) Exam

If you have studied the core psychiatric symptoms and illnesses, you will know a great deal about psychiatry. To specifically study for the clerkship or shelf exam, we recommend:

2–3 weeks before exam: Read this entire review book, taking notes.
10 days before exam: Read the notes you took during the rotation and the corresponding review book sections.
5 days before exam: Read this entire review book, concentrating on lists and mnemonics.
2 days before exam: Exercise, eat well, skim the book, and go to bed early.
1 day before exam: Exercise, eat well, review your notes and the mnemonics, and go to bed on time. Do not have any caffeine after 2 PM.

Other helpful studying strategies are discussed below.

STUDY WITH FRIENDS

Group studying can be very helpful. Other people may point out areas that you have not studied enough and may help you focus more effectively. If you tend to get distracted by other people in the room, limit this amount to less than half of your study time.

STUDY IN A BRIGHT ROOM

Find the room in your home or library that has the brightest light. This will help prevent you from falling asleep. If you don't have a bright light, obtain a halogen desk lamp or a light that simulates sunlight.

EAT LIGHT, BALANCED MEALS

Make sure your meals are balanced, with lean protein, fruits and vegetables, and fiber. A high-sugar, high-carbohydrate meal will give you an initial burst of energy for 1–2 hours, but then your blood sugar will quickly drop.

UTILIZE QUESTION BANKS AND/OR TAKE PRACTICE EXAMS

The purpose of practice exams is not just for the content that is contained in the questions, but the process of sitting for several hours and attempting to choose the best answer for each and every question.

POCKET CARDS

The "cards" on the following page contain information that is often helpful in psychiatry practice. We advise that you make a photocopy of these cards, cut them out, and carry them with you.

Mental Status Exam

Appearance/Behavior: Apparent age, attitude and cooperativeness, eye contact, posture, dress and hygiene, psychomotor status.

Speech: Rate, rhythm, volume, tone, articulation.

Mood: Patient's subjective emotional state—depressed, anxious, sad, angry, etc.

Affect: Objective emotional expression—euthymic, dysphoric, euphoric, appropriate (to stated mood), labile, full, constricted, flat, etc.

Thought process: Logical/linear, circumstantial, tangential, flight of ideas, looseness of association, thought blocking.

Thought content: Suicidal/homicidal ideation, delusions, ideas of reference, paranoia, obsessions, preoccupations, hyperreligiosity.

Perceptual disturbances: Hallucinations, illusions, derealization, depersonalization.

Cognition:

    Level of consciousness: Alert, sleepy, lethargic.
    Orientation: Person, place, date.
    Attention/Concentration: Serial 7s, spell "world" backwards.
    Abstract thought: Interpretation of proverbs, analogies.

    Memory:

        Registration: Immediate recall of three objects.
        Short term: Recall of objects after 5 minutes.
        Long term: Ask about verifiable personal information.
        Fund of knowledge: Current events.

Insight: Patient's awareness of his/her illness and need for treatment.

Judgment: Patient's ability to approach his/her problems in an appropriate manner.

Delirium

Characteristics: Acute onset, waxing/waning sensorium (worse at night), disorientation, inattention, impaired cognition, disorganized thinking, altered sleep-wake cycle, perceptual disorders (hallucinations, illusions).

(continued)

Etiology: Drugs (narcotics, benzodiazepines, anticholinergics (e.g., diphenhydramine), TCAs, steroids), EtOH withdrawal, metabolic (cardiac, respiratory, renal, hepatic, endocrine), infection, neurological causes (increased ICP, encephalitis, postictal, stroke).

Investigations:

Routine: CBC, chemistry panel, glucose, LFTs, TFTs, thiamine, folate, UA, urine. toxicology, CXR, vital signs.
Medium-yield: ABG, ECG (silent MI), ionized Ca^{2+}.
If above inconclusive: Head CT/MRI, EEG, LP.

Management: Identify/correct underlying cause, simplify Rx regimen, discontinue potentially offensive medications if possible, avoid benzodiazepines (except in EtOH withdrawal), create safe environment, provide reassurance/education, judiciously use antipsychotics for acute agitation.

Mini-Mental State Examination (MMSE)

Orientation (10):

What is the [year] [season] [date] [day] [month]? (1 pt. each)
Where are we [state] [county] [town] [hospital] [floor]?

Registration (3): Ask the patient to repeat three unrelated objects (1 pt. each on first attempt). If incomplete on first attempt, repeat up to six times (record number of trials).

Attention (5): Either serial 7s or spell "world" backwards (1 pt. for each correct letter or number).

Delayed recall (3): Ask patient to recall the three objects previously named (1 pt. each).

Language (9):

- Name two common objects, e.g., watch, pen (1 pt. each).
- Repeat the following sentence: "No ifs, ands, or buts" (1 pt.).
- Give patient blank paper. "Take it in your right hand, use both hands to fold it in half, and then put it on the floor" (1 pt. for each part correctly executed).
- Have patient read and follow: "Close your eyes" (1 pt.).
- Ask patient to write a sentence. The sentence must contain a subject and a verb; correct grammar and punctuation are not necessary (1 pt.).
- Ask the patient to copy the design. Each figure must have five sides, and two of the angles must intersect (1 pt.).

Mania ("DIG FAST")

Distractibility
Irritable mood/insomnia
Grandiosity
Flight of ideas
Agitation/increase in goal-directed activity
Speedy thoughts/speech
Thoughtlessness: seek pleasure without regard to consequences

Suicide Risk ("SAD PERSONS")

Sex—male
Age >60 years
Depression
Previous attempt
Ethanol/drug abuse
Rational thinking loss
Suicide in family
Organized plan/access
No support
Sickness

Major Depression ("SIG E. CAPS")

Sleep
Interest
Guilt
Energy
Concentration
Appetite
Psychomotor Δs
Suicidal ideation
    Hopelessness
    Helplessness
    Worthlessness

Drugs of Abuse

Drug	Intoxication	Withdrawal
Alcohol Benzodiazepines	Disinhibition, mood lability, incoordination, slurred speech, ataxia, blackouts (EtOH), respiratory depression	Tremulousness, hypertension, tachycardia, anxiety, psychomotor agitation, nausea, seizures, hallucinations, DTs (EtOH)
Barbiturates	Respiratory depression	Anxiety, seizures, delirium, life-threatening cardiovascular collapse

(continued)

Opioids	CNS depression, nausea, vomiting, sedation, decreased pain perception, decreased GI motility, pupil constriction, respiratory depression	Increased sympathetic activity, N/V, diarrhea, diaphoresis, rhinorrhea, piloerection, yawning, stomach cramps, myalgias, arthralgias, restlessness, anxiety, anorexia
Amphetamines Cocaine	Euphoria, increased attention span, aggressiveness, psychomotor agitation, pupil dilatation, hypertension, tachycardia, cardiac arrhythmias, psychosis, formication with cocaine	Post-use "crash": restlessness, headache, hunger, severe depression, irritability, insomnia/hypersomnia, strong psychological craving
PCP	Belligerence, impulsiveness, psychomotor agitation, vertical/horizontal nystagmus, hyperthermia, tachycardia, ataxia, psychosis, homicidality	May have recurrence of symptoms due to reabsorption in GI tract
LSD	Altered perceptual states (hallucinations, distortions of time and space), elevation of mood, "bad trips" (panic reaction), flashbacks (reexperience of the sensations in absence of drug use)	
Cannabis	Euphoria, anxiety, paranoia, slowed time, social withdrawal, increased appetite, dry mouth, tachycardia, amotivational syndrome	
Nicotine/Caffeine	Restlessness, insomnia, anxiety, anorexia	Irritability, lethargy, headache, increased appetite, weight gain

First Aid for the Psychiatry Clerkship, 4e; copyright © 2015 McGraw-Hill. All rights reserved.

Psychiatric Emergencies

Delirium Tremens (DTs):
- Typically within 2–4 days after cessation of EtOH but may occur later.
- Delirium, agitation, fever, autonomic hyperactivity, auditory and visual hallucinations.
- Treat aggressively with benzodiazepines and hydration.

Neuroleptic Malignant Syndrome (NMS):
- Fever, rigidity, autonomic instability, clouding of consciousness, elevated WBC/CPK.
- Withhold neuroleptics, hydrate, consider dantrolene, and/or bromocriptine.
- Idiosyncratic, time-limited reaction.

Serotonin Syndrome:
- Precipitated by use of two drugs with serotonin-enhancing properties (e.g., MAOI + SSRI).
- Altered mental status, fever, agitation, tremor, myoclonus, hyperreflexia, ataxia, incoordination, diaphoresis, shivering, diarrhea.
- Discontinue offending agents, benzodiazepines, consider cyproheptadine.

Tyramine Reaction/Hypertensive Crisis:
- Precipitated by ingestion of tyramine-containing foods while on MAOIs.
- Hypertension, headache, neck stiffness, sweating, nausea, vomiting, visual problems. Most serious consequences are stroke and possibly death.
- Treat with nitroprusside or phentolamine.

Acute Dystonia:
- Early, sudden onset of muscle spasm: eyes, tongue, jaw, neck; may lead to laryngospasm requiring intubation.
- Treat with benztropine (Cogentin) or diphenhydramine (Benadryl).
- If clinically appropriate, reduce the dose, discontinue the medication, or switch to another agent.

Lithium Toxicity:
- May occur at any Li level (usually >1.5).
- Nausea, vomiting, slurred speech, ataxia, incoordination, myoclonus, hyperreflexia, seizures, nephrogenic diabetes insipidus, delirium, coma.
- Discontinue Li, hydrate aggressively, consider hemodialysis.

Tricyclic Antidepressant (TCA) Toxicity:
- Primarily anticholinergic effects, cardiac conduction disturbances, hypotension, respiratory depression, agitation, hallucinations, seizures.
- Classic ECG finding is QRS > 100 msec.
- Sodium bicarbonate, activated charcoal, cathartics, supportive treatment.
- Discontinue the medication.

NOTES

CHAPTER 2

EXAMINATION AND DIAGNOSIS

History and Mental Status Examination	12
INTERVIEWING	12
TAKING THE HISTORY	13
MENTAL STATUS EXAMINATION	13
BEDSIDE COGNITIVE TESTING	17
Interviewing Skills	17
GENERAL APPROACHES TO TYPES OF PATIENTS	17
Diagnosis and Classification	19
DIAGNOSIS AS PER DSM-5	19
Diagnostic Testing	19
INTELLIGENCE TESTS	19
OBJECTIVE PERSONALITY ASSESSMENT TESTS	19
PROJECTIVE (PERSONALITY) ASSESSMENT TESTS	20

WARDS TIP

The history of present illness (HPI) should include information about the current episode, including symptoms, duration, context, stressors, and impairment in function.

History and Mental Status Examination

INTERVIEWING

Making the Patient Comfortable

The initial interview is of utmost importance to the psychiatrist. With practice, you will develop your own style and learn how to adapt the interview to the individual patient. In general, start the interview by asking open-ended questions. Carefully note how the patient responds, as this is critical information for the mental status exam. Consider preparing for the interview by writing down the subheadings of the exam (see Figure 2-1). Find a safe and private area to conduct the interview. Use closed-ended questions to obtain the remaining pertinent information. During the first interview, the psychiatrist must establish a meaningful rapport with the patient in order to get accurate and pertinent information. This requires that the questions be asked in a quiet, comfortable setting so that the patient is at ease. The patient

```
Date and Location:

Identifying Patient Data:



Chief Complaint:                          Past Medical History:
History of Present Illness:
                                          Allergies:

Past Psychiatric History:                 Current Meds:
First contact:
                                          Developmental History:
Diagnosis:
Prior hospitalizations:
                                          Relationships (children/marital status):
Suicide attempts:
Outpatient treatment:
                                          Education:
Med trials:
                                          Work History:

Substance History:                        Military History:
                                          Housing:
Smoking:                                  Income:
Family Psychiatric and Medical History:   Religion:


Legal History:
```

FIGURE 2-1. Psychiatric history outline

should feel that the psychiatrist is interested, nonjudgmental, and compassionate. In psychiatry, the history is the most important factor in formulating a diagnosis and treatment plan.

TAKING THE HISTORY

The psychiatric history follows a similar format as the history for other types of patients. It should include the following:

- Identifying data: The patient's name, gender, age, race, marital status.
- Chief complaint (use the patient's own words): If called as a consultant, list reason for the consult.
- Sources of information.
- History of present illness (HPI):
  - *The 4 Ps:* The patient's psychosocial and environmental conditions *predisposing to, precipitating, perpetuating,* and *protecting* against the current episode.
  - The patient's support system (whom the patient lives with, distance and level of contact with friends and relatives).
  - Neurovegetative symptoms (quality of sleep, appetite, energy, psychomotor retardation/activation, concentration).
  - Suicidal ideation/homicidal ideation.
  - How work and relationship have been affected (for most diagnoses in the *Diagnostic and Statistical Manual of Mental Disorders*, 5th edition [DSM-5] there is a criterion that specifies that symptoms must cause clinically significant distress or impairment in social, occupational, or other important areas of functioning).
  - Psychotic symptoms (e.g., auditory and visual hallucinations, delusions).
  - Establish a baseline of mental health:
    - Patient's level of functioning when "well."
    - Goals (outpatient setting).
- Past psychiatric history (include as applicable: history of suicide attempts, history of self-harm [e.g., cutting, burning oneself], information about previous episodes, other psychiatric disorders in remission, medication trials, past psychiatric hospitalizations, current psychiatrist).
- Substance history (age of first use, history of withdrawal/delirium tremens, longest period of sobriety, history of intravenous drug use, participation in outpatient or inpatient drug rehab programs).
- Medical history (ask specifically about head trauma, seizures, pregnancy status).
- Family psychiatric and medical history (include substance use, suicides, and response to specific psychotropic agents as patient may respond similarly).
- Medications (ask about supplements and over-the-counter (OTC) medications, as well as compliance).
- Allergies: Clarify if it was a true allergy or an adverse drug event (e.g., abdominal pain).
- Developmental/Social history: Achieved developmental milestones on time, friends in school, history of trauma or abuse, performance academically. Also include income source, employment, education, place of residence, who they live with, number of children, support system, religious affiliation and beliefs, legal history, and amount of exercise.

MENTAL STATUS EXAMINATION

This is analogous to performing a physical exam in other areas of medicine. It is the nuts and bolts of the psychiatric exam. It should describe

WARDS TIP

If you are seeing the patient in the ER, make sure to ask how they got to the ER (police, bus, walk-in, family member) and look to see what time they were triaged. For all initial evaluations, ask why the patient is seeking treatment *today* as opposed to any other day.

WARDS TIP

When taking a substance history, remember to ask about caffeine and nicotine use. If a heavy smoker is hospitalized and does not have access to nicotine replacement therapy, nicotine withdrawal may cause anxiety and agitation.

KEY FACT

Importance of asking about OTC use: Nonsteroidal anti-inflammatory drugs (NSAIDs) can ↓ lithium excretion → ↑ lithium concentrations (exceptions may be sulindac and aspirin).

WARDS TIP

Psychomotor retardation, which refers to the slowness of voluntary and involuntary movements, may also be referred to as hypokinesia or bradykinesia. The term akinesia is used in extreme cases where absence of movement is observed.

KEY FACT

Automatisms are spontaneous, involuntary movements that occur during an altered state of consciousness and can range from purposeful to disorganized.

WARDS TIP

A hallmark of pressured speech is that it is usually uninterruptible and the patient is compelled to continue speaking.

WARDS TIP

To assess mood, ask, "How are you feeling today?" It can also be helpful to have patients rate their stated mood on a scale of 1–10.

WARDS TIP

A patient who remains expressionless and monotone even when discussing extremely sad or happy moments in his life has a *flat* affect.

KEY FACT

An example of inappropriate affect is a patient's laughing when being told he has a serious illness.

the patient in as much detail as possible. The mental status exam assesses the following:

- Appearance/Behavior
- Speech
- Mood/Affect
- Thought process
- Thought content
- Perceptual disturbances
- Cognition
- Insight
- Judgment/Impulse control

The mental status exam tells only about the mental status at that moment; it can change every hour or every day, etc.

Appearance/Behavior

- *Appearance:* Gender, age (looks older/younger than stated age), type of clothing, hygiene (including smelling of alcohol, urine, feces), posture, grooming, physical abnormalities, tattoos, body piercings. Take specific notice of the following, which may be clues for possible diagnoses:
  - Pupil size: Drug intoxication/withdrawal.
  - Bruises in hidden areas: ↑ suspicion for abuse.
  - Needle marks/tracks: Drug use.
  - Eroding of tooth enamel: Eating disorders (from vomiting).
  - Superficial cuts on arms: Self-harm.
- *Behavior:* Attitude (cooperative, seductive, flattering, charming, eager to please, entitled, controlling, uncooperative, hostile, guarded, critical, antagonistic, childish), mannerisms, tics, eye contact, activity level, psychomotor retardation/activation, akathisia, automatisms, catatonia, choreoathetoid movements, compulsions, dystonias, tremor.

Speech

Rate (pressured, slowed, regular), rhythm (i.e., prosody), articulation (dysarthria, stuttering), accent/dialect, volume/modulation (loudness or softness), tone, long or short latency of speech.

Mood

Mood is the emotion that the patient tells you he/she feels, often in quotations.

Affect

Affect is an assessment of how the patient's mood appears to the examiner, including the amount and range of emotional expression. It is described with the following dimensions:

- *Type of affect:* Euthymic, euphoric, neutral, dysphoric.
- *Range* describes the depth and range of the feelings shown. Parameters: flat (none)—blunted (shallow)—constricted (limited)—full (average)—intense (more than normal).
- *Motility* describes how quickly a person appears to shift emotional states. Parameters: sluggish—supple—labile.
- *Appropriateness to content* describes whether the affect is congruent with the subject of conversation or stated mood. Parameters: appropriate—not appropriate.

Thought Process

The patient's form of thinking—how he or she uses language and puts ideas together. It describes whether the patient's thoughts are logical, meaningful, and goal directed. It does not comment on *what* the patient thinks, only *how* the patient expresses his or her thoughts.

- **Logical/Linear/Goal-directed:** Answers to questions and conversation clear and follows a logical sequence.
- **Circumstantiality** is when the point of the conversation is eventually reached but with overinclusion of trivial or irrelevant details.

Examples of thought disorders include:

- **Tangentiality:** Can follow conversation but point never reached or question never answered.
- **Loosening of associations:** No logical connection from one thought to another.
- **Flight of ideas:** Thoughts change abruptly from one idea to another, usually accompanied by rapid/pressured speech.
- **Neologisms:** Made-up words.
- **Word salad:** Incoherent collection of words.
- **Clang associations:** Word connections due to phonetics rather than actual meaning. "My car is red. I've been in bed. It hurts my head."
- **Thought blocking:** Abrupt cessation of communication before the idea is finished.

Thought Content

Describes the types of ideas expressed by the patient. Examples of disorders:

- **Poverty of thought versus overabundance:** Too few versus too many ideas expressed.
- **Delusions:** Fixed, false beliefs that are not shared by the person's culture and remain despite evidence to the contrary. Delusions are classified as bizarre (impossible to be true) or nonbizarre (at least possible).
- **Suicidal and homicidal ideation:** Ask if the patient feels like harming himself/herself or others. Identify if the plan is well formulated. Ask if the patient has an intent (i.e., if released right now, would he/she go and kill himself/herself or harm others?). Ask if the patient has means to kill himself/herself (firearms in the house/multiple prescription bottles).
- **Phobias:** Persistent, irrational fears.
- **Obsessions:** Repetitive, intrusive thoughts.

Perceptual Disturbances

- *Hallucinations:* Sensory perceptions that occur in the absence of an actual stimulus.
  - Describe the sensory modality: Auditory (most common), visual, gustatory, olfactory, or tactile.
  - Describe the details (e.g., auditory hallucinations may be ringing, humming, whispers, or voices speaking clear words). Command auditory hallucinations are voices that instruct the patient to do something.
  - Ask if the hallucination is experienced only while falling asleep (hypnagogic hallucination) or upon awakening (hypnopompic hallucination).
- *Illusions:* Inaccurate perception of existing sensory stimuli (e.g., wall appears as if it's moving).
- *Derealization/Depersonalization:* The experience of feeling detached from one's surroundings/mental processes.

WARDS TIP

A patient who is laughing one second and crying the next has a *labile* affect.

KEY FACT

Examples of delusions:
- *Grandeur*—belief that one has special powers or is someone important (Jesus, President).
- *Paranoid*—belief that one is being persecuted.
- *Reference*—belief that some event is uniquely related to patient (e.g., a TV show character is sending patient messages).
- *Thought broadcasting*—belief that one's thoughts can be heard by others.
- *Religious*—conventional beliefs exaggerated (e.g., God wants me to be the Messiah).
- *Somatic*—false belief concerning body image (e.g., I have cancer).

WARDS TIP

The following question can help screen for obsessions: Do you think and/or worry about checking, cleaning, or counting on a repetitive basis?

WARDS TIP

An auditory hallucination that instructs a patient to harm himself or others is an important risk factor for suicide or homicide.

WARDS TIP

Alcoholic hallucinosis refers to hallucinations (usually auditory, although visual and tactile may occur) that occur either during or after a period of heavy alcohol consumption. Patients usually are aware that these hallucinations are not real. In contrast to delirium tremens (DTs), there is no clouding of sensorium and vital signs are normal.

KEY FACT

You can roughly assess a patient's intellectual functioning by utilizing the *proverb interpretation* and *vocabulary* strategies. Proverb interpretation is helpful in assessing whether a patient has difficulty with abstraction. Being able to define a particular vocabulary word correctly and appropriately use it in a sentence reflects a person's intellectual capacity.

WARDS TIP

To test ability to abstract, ask:
1. Similarities: How are an apple and orange alike? (Normal answer: "They are fruits." *Concrete* answer: "They are round.")
2. Proverb testing: What is meant by the phrase, "You can't judge a book by its cover?" (Normal answer: "You can't judge people just by how they look." *Concrete* answer: "Books have different covers.")

Cognition

- **Consciousness:** Patient's level of awareness; possible range includes: alert—drowsy—lethargic—stuporous—comatose.
- **Orientation:** To person, place, and time.
- **Calculation:** Ability to add/subtract.
- **Memory:**
    - Immediate (registration)—dependent on attention/concentration and can be tested by asking a patient to repeat several digits or words.
    - Recent (short-term memory)—events within the past few minutes, hours, or days.
    - Remote memory (long-term memory).
- **Fund of knowledge:** Level of knowledge in the context of the patient's culture and education (e.g., Who is the president? Who was Picasso?).
- **Attention/Concentration:** Ability to subtract serial 7s from 100 or to spell "world" backward.
- **Reading/Writing:** Simple sentences (must make sure the patient is literate first).
- **Abstract concepts:** Ability to explain similarities between objects and understand the meaning of simple proverbs.

Insight

Insight is the patient's level of awareness and understanding of his or her problem. Problems with insight include complete denial of illness or blaming it on something else. Insight can be described as full, partial/limited, or minimal.

Judgment

Judgment is the patient's ability to understand the outcome of his or her actions and use this awareness in decision making; it is best determined from information from the HPI and recent behavior (e.g., how a patient was brought to treatment or medication compliance). Judgment can be described as excellent, good, fair, or poor.

> Mrs. W is a 52-year-old Asian-American woman who arrives at the emergency room reporting that her deceased husband of 25 years told her that he would be waiting for her there. To meet him, she drove nonstop for 22 hours from a nearby state. She claims that her husband is a famous preacher and that she, too, has a mission from God. Although she does not specify the details of her mission, she says that she was given the ability to stop time until her mission is completed. She reports experiencing high levels of energy despite not sleeping for 22 hours. She also reports that she has a history of psychiatric hospitalizations but refuses to provide further information.
>
> While obtaining her history you perform a mental status exam. Her **appearance** is that of a woman who looks older than her stated age. She is obese and unkempt. There is no evidence of tattoos or piercings. She has tousled hair and is dressed in a mismatched flowered skirt and a red T-shirt. Upon her arrival at the emergency room, her **behavior** is demanding, as she insists that you let her husband know that she has arrived. She then becomes irate and proceeds to yell, banging her head against the wall. She screams, "Stop hiding him from me!" She is uncooperative with redirection and is guarded during the remainder of the interview. Her eye contact is poor as she is looking around the room.

Her **psychomotor activity** is agitated. Her **speech** is loud and pressured, with a foreign accent.

She reports that her **mood** is "angry," and her **affect** as observed during the interview is labile and irritable.

Her **thought process** includes flight of ideas. Her **thought content** is significant for delusions of grandeur and thought broadcasting, as evidenced by her refusing to answer most questions claiming that you are able to know what she is thinking. She denies suicidal or homicidal ideation. She expresses **disturbances in perception** as she admits to frequent auditory hallucinations without commands.

She is uncooperative with formal **cognitive** testing, but you notice that she is oriented to place and person. However, she erroneously states that it is 2005. Her attention and concentration are notably impaired, as she appears distracted and frequently needs questions repeated. Her **insight, judgment, and impulse control** are determined to be poor.

You decide to admit Mrs. W to the inpatient psychiatric unit in order to allow for comprehensive diagnostic evaluation, the opportunity to obtain collateral information from her prior hospitalizations, safety monitoring, medical workup for possible reversible causes of her symptoms, and psychopharmacological treatment.

BEDSIDE COGNITIVE TESTING

The Montreal Cognitive Assessment (MOCA)

The MOCA is a simple, brief test used to assess gross cognitive functioning. The test and its instructions are available online (Figure 2-2). The areas tested include:

- Orientation (to person, place, and time).
- Memory (immediate—repeating five words; and recent—recalling the words 5 minutes later).
- Attention (serial 7s, tapping hand with certain letters, repeating digits).
- Language (naming, repetition, fluency).
- Abstraction (e.g., saying how a "train" and "bicycle" are alike).
- Visuospatial ability/executive functioning (trail making task, cube copying, clock drawing).

The Mini-Mental State Examination (MMSE)

The MMSE is another test of cognition that can be performed in a few minutes at the bedside. Unlike the MOCA, the MMSE is copyright protected.

Interviewing Skills

GENERAL APPROACHES TO TYPES OF PATIENTS

Violent Patient

Do not interview a potentially violent patient alone. Inform staff of your whereabouts. Know if there are accessible panic buttons. To assess violence

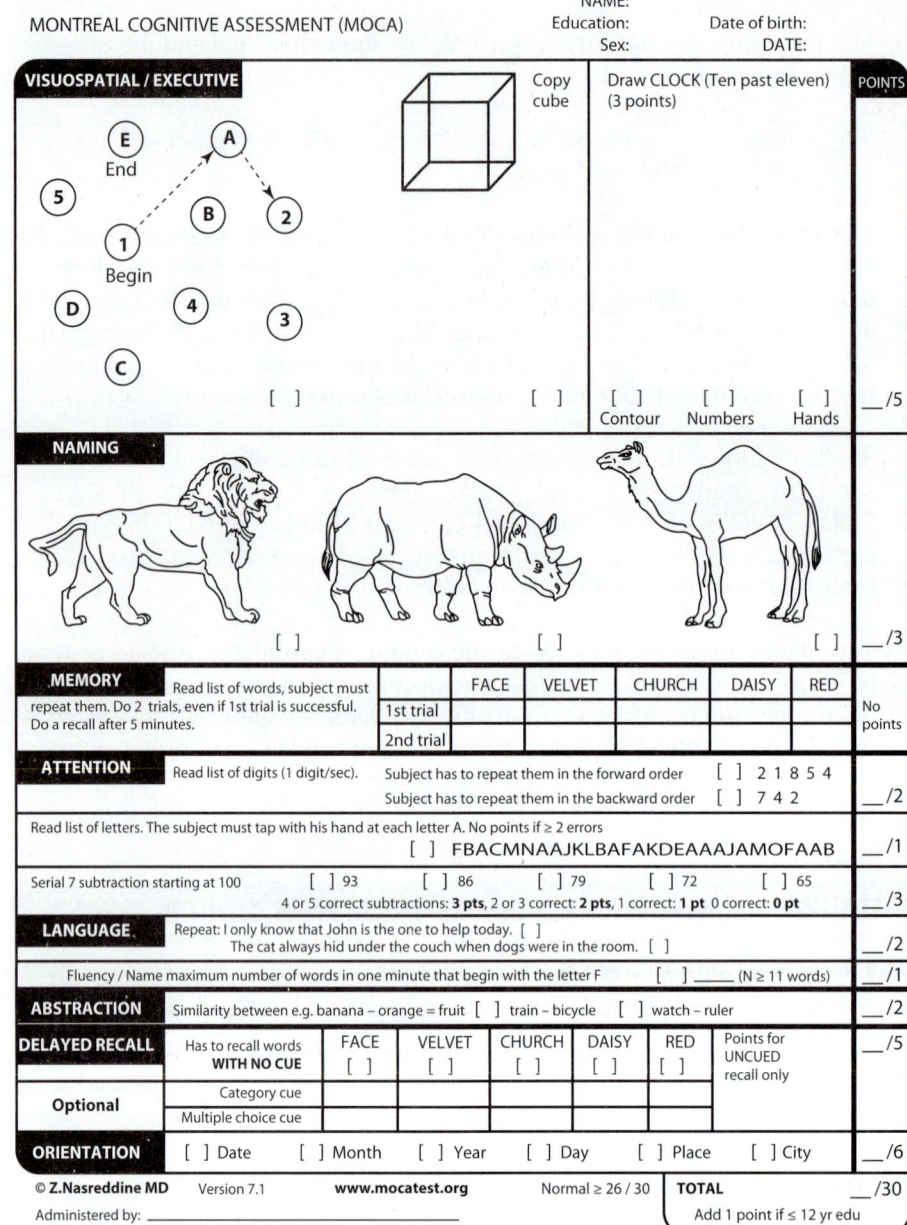

FIGURE 2-2. Montreal Cognitive Assessment Test (MoCA). Copyright © Z. Nasreddine MD. Reproduced with permission. Copies are available at www.mocatest.org

KEY FACT

A prior history of violence is the most important predictor of future violence.

or homicidality, one can simply ask, "Do you feel like you want to hurt someone or that you might hurt someone?" If the patient expresses imminent threats against specific friends, family, or others, the doctor must notify potential victims and/or protection agencies (Tarasoff Rule).

Delusional Patient

Although the psychiatrist should not directly challenge a delusion or insist that it is untrue, he/she should not imply he believes it either. He/she should simply acknowledge that he/she understands that the *patient believes* the delusion is true.

Depressed Patient

A depressed patient may be skeptical that he or she can be helped. It is important to offer reassurance that he or she can improve with appropriate therapy. Inquiring about suicidal thoughts is crucial; a feeling of hopelessness, substance use, and/or a history of prior suicide attempts reveal an ↑ risk for suicide. If the patient is actively planning or contemplating suicide, he or she should be hospitalized or otherwise protected.

Diagnosis and Classification

DIAGNOSIS AS PER DSM-5

The American Psychiatric Association (APA) uses a criterion-based system for diagnoses. Criteria and codes for each diagnosis are outlined in the DSM-5.

WARDS TIP

In assessing suicidality, do not simply ask, "Do you want to hurt yourself?" because this does not directly address suicidality (he/she may plan on dying in a painless way). Ask directly about killing self or suicide. If contemplating suicide, ask the patient if he/she has a plan of how to do it and if he/she has intent; a detailed plan, intent, and the means to accomplish it suggest a serious threat.

Diagnostic Testing

INTELLIGENCE TESTS

Aspects of intelligence include memory, logical reasoning, ability to assimilate factual knowledge, and understanding of abstract concepts.

Intelligence Quotient (IQ)

IQ is a test of intelligence with a mean of 100 and a standard deviation of 15. These scores are adjusted for age. An IQ of 100 signifies that mental age equals chronological age and corresponds to the 50th percentile in intellectual ability for the general population.

Intelligence tests assess cognitive function by evaluating comprehension, fund of knowledge, math skills, vocabulary, picture assembly, and other verbal and performance skills. Two common tests are:

Wechsler Adult Intelligence Scale (WAIS):

- Most common test for ages 16–90.
- Assesses overall intellectual functioning.
- Four index scores: Verbal comprehension, perceptual reasoning, working memory, processing speed.

Wechsler Intelligence Scale for Children (WISC): Tests intellectual ability in patients ages 6–16.

OBJECTIVE PERSONALITY ASSESSMENT TESTS

These tests are questions with standardized-answer format that are objectively scored. The following is an example:

Minnesota Multiphasic Personality Inventory (MMPI-2)

- Tests personality for different pathologies and behavioral patterns.
- Most commonly used.

KEY FACT

The Minnesota Multiphasic Personality Inventory (MMPI) is an objective psychological test that is used to assess a person's personality and identify psychopathologies. The mean score for each scale is 50 and the standard deviation is 10.

WARDS TIP

IQ Chart
Very superior: >130
Superior: 120–129
High average: 110–119
Average: 90–109
Low average: 80–89
Borderline: 70–79
Extremely low (intellectual disability): <70

PROJECTIVE (PERSONALITY) ASSESSMENT TESTS

Projective tests have no structured-response format. The tests often ask for interpretation of ambiguous stimuli. Examples are:

Thematic Apperception Test (TAT)

- Test taker creates stories based on pictures of people in various situations.
- Used to evaluate motivations behind behaviors.

Rorschach Test

- Interpretation of inkblots.
- Used to identify thought disorders and defense mechanisms.

CHAPTER 3
PSYCHOTIC DISORDERS

Psychosis	22
Delusions	22
Perceptual Disturbances	22
Differential Diagnosis of Psychosis	22
Psychotic Disorder Due to Another Medical Condition	23
Substance/Medication-Induced Psychotic Disorder	23
Schizophrenia	23
Positive, Negative, and Cognitive Symptoms	24
Three Phases	24
Diagnosis of Schizophrenia	24
Psychiatric Exam of Patients with Schizophrenia	26
Epidemiology	26
Downward Drift	26
Pathophysiology of Schizophrenia: The Dopamine Hypothesis	26
Other Neurotransmitter Abnormalities Implicated in Schizophrenia	27
Prognostic Factors	27
Treatment	28
Schizophreniform Disorder	29
Schizoaffective Disorder	30
Brief Psychotic Disorder	30
Delusional Disorder	31
Culture-Specific Psychoses	32
Comparing Time Courses and Prognoses of Psychotic Disorders	32
Quick and Easy Distinguishing Features	32

WARDS TIP

Psychosis is exemplified by delusions, hallucinations, or severe disorganization of thought/behavior.

Psychosis

Psychosis is a general term used to describe a distorted perception of reality. Poor reality testing may be accompanied by delusions, perceptual disturbances (illusions or hallucinations), and/or disorganized thinking/behavior. Psychosis can be a symptom of schizophrenia, mania, depression, delirium, and major neurocognitive disorder (i.e., dementia), and it can be substance or medication-induced.

DELUSIONS

Delusions are fixed, false beliefs that persist despite evidence to the contrary and that do not make sense within the context of an individual's cultural background.

They can be categorized as either bizarre or nonbizarre. A *nonbizarre* delusion is a false belief that is plausible but is not true. Example: "The neighbors are spying on me by reading my e-mail." A *bizarre* delusion is a false belief that is impossible. Example: "Aliens are spying on me through a Wi-Fi connection in my brain."

Delusions can also be categorized by theme:

- **Delusions of persecution/paranoid delusions:** Irrational belief that one is being persecuted. Example: "The Central Intelligence Agency (CIA) is monitoring me and tapped my cell phone."
- **Ideas of reference:** Belief that cues in the external environment are uniquely related to the individual. Example: "The TV characters are speaking directly to me."
- **Delusions of control:** Includes **thought broadcasting** (belief that one's thoughts can be heard by others) and **thought insertion** (belief that outside thoughts are being placed in one's head).
- **Delusions of grandeur:** Belief that one has special powers beyond those of a normal person. Example: "I am the all-powerful son of God and I shall bring down my wrath on you if I don't get my way."
- **Delusions of guilt:** Belief that one is guilty or responsible for something. Example: "I am responsible for all the world's wars."
- **Somatic delusions:** Belief that one has a certain illness or health condition. Example: A patient believing she is pregnant despite negative pregnancy tests and ultrasounds.

PERCEPTUAL DISTURBANCES

- **Illusion:** Misinterpretation of an existing sensory stimulus (such as mistaking a shadow for an evil spirit).
- **Hallucination:** Sensory perception without an actual external stimulus.
    - **Auditory:** Most commonly exhibited by schizophrenic patients.
    - **Visual:** Occurs, but less common in schizophrenia. May accompany drug intoxication, drug and alcohol withdrawal, or delirium.
    - **Olfactory:** Usually an aura associated with epilepsy.
    - **Tactile:** Usually secondary to drug use or alcohol withdrawal.

WARDS TIP

Auditory hallucinations that directly tell the patient to perform certain acts are called *command hallucinations*.

DIFFERENTIAL DIAGNOSIS OF PSYCHOSIS

- Psychotic disorder due to another medical condition.
- Substance/Medication-induced psychotic disorder.

- Delirium/Major neurocognitive disorder (dementia).
- Bipolar disorder, manic/mixed episode.
- Major depression with psychotic features.
- Brief psychotic disorder.
- Schizophrenia.
- Schizophreniform disorder.
- Schizoaffective disorder.
- Delusional disorder.

PSYCHOTIC DISORDER DUE TO ANOTHER MEDICAL CONDITION

Other Medical causes of psychosis include:

1. *Central nervous system (CNS) disease* (cerebrovascular disease, multiple sclerosis, neoplasm, Alzheimer disease, Parkinson disease, Huntington disease, tertiary syphilis, epilepsy [often temporal lobe], encephalitis, prion disease, neurosarcoidosis, AIDS).
2. *Endocrinopathies* (Addison/Cushing disease, hyper/hypothyroidism, hyper/hypocalcemia, hypopituitarism).
3. *Nutritional/Vitamin deficiency states* (B12, folate, niacin).
4. *Other* (connective tissue disease [systemic lupus erythematosus, temporal arteritis], porphyria).

DSM-5 criteria for psychotic disorder due to another medical condition include:

- Prominent hallucinations or delusions.
- Symptoms do not occur only during an episode of delirium.
- Evidence from history, physical, or lab data to support another medical cause (i.e., not a primary psychiatric disorder).

SUBSTANCE/MEDICATION-INDUCED PSYCHOTIC DISORDER

Prescription medications that may cause psychosis in some patients include anesthetics, antimicrobials, corticosteroids, antiparkinsonian agents, anticonvulsants, antihistamines, anticholinergics, antihypertensives, nonsteroidal anti-inflammatory drugs (NSAIDs), digitalis, methylphenidate, and chemotherapeutic agents. Substances such as alcohol, cocaine, hallucinogens (LSD, ecstasy), cannabis, benzodiazepines, barbiturates, inhalants, and phencyclidine (PCP) can cause psychosis, either during intoxication or withdrawal.

DSM-5 Criteria

- Hallucinations and/or delusions.
- Symptoms do not occur only during episode of delirium.
- Evidence from history, physical, or lab data to support a medication or substance-induced cause.
- Disturbance is not better accounted for by a psychotic disorder that is not substance/medication-induced.

Schizophrenia

A 24-year-old male graduate student without prior medical or psychiatric history is reported by his mother to have been very anxious over the past 9 months, with increasing concern that people are watching him. He now claims to "hear voices" telling him what must be

WARDS TIP

It's important to be able to distinguish between a delusion, illusion, and hallucination. A delusion is a fixed, false belief, an illusion is a misinterpretation of an external stimulus, and a hallucination is perception in the absence of an external stimulus.

WARDS TIP

Elderly, medically ill patients who present with psychotic symptoms such as hallucinations, confusion, or paranoia should be carefully evaluated for delirium, which is a far more common finding in this population.

WARDS TIP

To make the diagnosis of schizophrenia, a patient must have symptoms of the disease for at least 6 months.

> done to "fix the country." *Important workup?* Comprehensive metabolic panel, urine drug screen, thyroid-stimulating hormone (TSH), HIV testing. Consider brain imaging. *Likely diagnosis? If workup is unremarkable,* schizophrenia. *Next step?* Antipsychotics.

Schizophrenia is a psychiatric disorder characterized by a constellation of abnormalities in thinking, emotion, and behavior. There is no single symptom that is pathognomonic, and there is a heterogeneous clinical presentation. Schizophrenia is typically chronic, with significant psychosocial and medical consequences to the patient.

POSITIVE, NEGATIVE, AND COGNITIVE SYMPTOMS

In general, the symptoms of schizophrenia are broken up into three categories:

- **Positive symptoms:** Hallucinations, delusions, bizarre behavior, disorganized speech. These tend to respond more robustly to antipsychotic medications.
- **Negative symptoms:** Flat or blunted affect, anhedonia, apathy, alogia, and lack of interest in socialization. These symptoms are comparatively more often treatment resistant and contribute significantly to the social isolation and impaired function of schizophrenic patients.
- **Cognitive symptoms:** Impairments in attention, executive function, and working memory. These symptoms may **lead to** poor work and school performance.

KEY FACT

Think of positive symptoms as things that are ADDED onto normal behavior. Think of negative symptoms as things that are SUBTRACTED or missing from normal behavior.

THREE PHASES

Symptoms of schizophrenia often present in the following three phases:

1. **Prodromal:** Decline in functioning that precedes the first psychotic episode. The patient may become socially withdrawn and irritable. He or she may have physical complaints, declining school/work performance, and/or newfound interest in religion or the occult.
2. **Psychotic:** Perceptual disturbances, delusions, and disordered thought process/content.
3. **Residual:** Occurs following an episode of active psychosis. It is marked by mild hallucinations or delusions, social withdrawal, and negative symptoms.

WARDS TIP

Stereotyped movement, bizarre posturing, and muscle rigidity are examples of catatonia, a syndrome which can be seen in schizophrenia, depression, bipolar disorder, and other psychiatric conditions.

DIAGNOSIS OF SCHIZOPHRENIA

DSM-5 Criteria

- *Two or more* of the following must be present for at least *1 month:*
    1. Delusions.
    2. Hallucinations.
    3. Disorganized speech.
    4. Grossly disorganized or catatonic behavior.
    5. Negative symptoms.
    Note: At least one must be **1, 2,** or **3**.
- Must cause significant social, occupational, or functional (self-care) deterioration.

WARDS TIP

The 5 A's of schizophrenia (negative symptoms):
1. Anhedonia
2. Affect (flat)
3. Alogia (poverty of speech)
4. Avolition (apathy)
5. Attention (poor)

- Duration of illness for at least 6 months (including prodromal or residual periods in which the above full criteria may not be met).
- Symptoms not due to effects of a substance or another medical condition.

Mr. Torres is a 21-year-old man who is brought to the ER by his mother after he began talking about "aliens" who were trying to steal his soul. Mr. Torres reports that aliens leave messages for him by arranging sticks outside his home and sometimes send thoughts into his mind. On exam, he is guarded and often stops talking while in the middle of expressing a thought. Mr. Torres appears anxious and frequently scans the room for aliens, which he thinks may have followed him to the hospital. He denies any plan to harm himself, but admits that the aliens sometimes want him to throw himself in front of a car, "as this will change the systems that belong under us."

The patient's mother reports that he began expressing these ideas a few months ago, but they have become more severe in the last few weeks. She reports that during the past year, he has become isolated from his peers, frequently talks to himself, and has stopped going to community college. He has also spent most of his time reading science fiction books and creating devices that will prevent aliens from hurting him. She reports that she is concerned because the patient's father, who left while the patient was a child, exhibited similar symptoms many years ago and has spent most of his life in psychiatric hospitals.

What is Mr. Torres's most likely diagnosis? What differential diagnoses should be considered?

Mr. Torres's most likely diagnosis is schizophrenia. He exhibits delusional ideas that are bizarre and paranoid in nature. He also reports the presence of frequent auditory hallucinations and disturbances in thought process that include thought blocking. Although the patient's mother reports that his psychotic symptoms began "a few months ago," the patient has exhibited social and occupational dysfunction during the last year. Mr. Torres quit school, became isolated, and has been responding to internal stimuli since that time. In addition, his father appears to also suffer from a psychotic disorder. In this case, it appears that the disorder has been present for more than 6 months. However, if this is unclear, the diagnosis of schizophreniform disorder should be made instead.

The differential diagnosis should also include schizoaffective disorder, medication/substance-induced psychotic disorder, psychotic disorder due to another medical condition, and mood disorder with psychotic features.

What would be appropriate steps in the acute management of this patient?

Treatment should include inpatient hospitalization in order to provide a safe environment, with monitoring of suicidal ideation secondary to his psychosis. Routine laboratory tests, including a urine or serum drug screen, should be undertaken. The patient should begin treatment with antipsychotic medication while closely being monitored for potential side effects.

WARDS TIP

Echolalia—repeats words or phrases
EchoPRAxia—mimics behavior (PRActices behavior)

PSYCHIATRIC EXAM OF PATIENTS WITH SCHIZOPHRENIA

The *typical* findings in schizophrenic patients include:

- Disheveled appearance.
- Flat affect.
- Disorganized thought process.
- Intact procedural memory and orientation.
- Auditory hallucinations.
- Paranoid delusions.
- Ideas of reference.
- Lack of insight into their disease.

Keep in mind that schizophrenia can have a very heterogeneous presentation—patients may have schizophrenia without a disheveled appearance or clear negative symptoms.

KEY FACT

Brief psychotic disorder lasts for <1 month. Schizophreniform disorder can last between 1 and 6 months. Schizophrenia lasts for >6 months.

EPIDEMIOLOGY

- Schizophrenia affects approximately 0.3–0.7% of people over their lifetime.
- Men and women are equally affected but have different presentations and outcomes:
  - Men tend to present in early to mid-20s.
  - Women present in late 20s.
  - Men tend to have more negative symptoms and poorer outcome compared to women.
- Schizophrenia rarely presents before age 15 or after age 55.
- There is a strong genetic predisposition:
  - Fifty percent concordance rate among monozygotic twins.
  - Forty percent risk of inheritance if both parents have schizophrenia.
  - Twelve percent risk if one first-degree relative is affected.
- Substance use is comorbid in many patients with schizophrenia. The most commonly abused substance is nicotine (>50%), followed by alcohol, cannabis, and cocaine.
- Post-psychotic depression is the phenomenon of schizophrenic patients developing a major depressive episode after resolution of their psychotic symptoms.

KEY FACT

People born in late winter and early spring have a higher incidence of schizophrenia for unknown reasons. (One theory involves seasonal variation in viral infections, particularly second-trimester exposure to influenza virus.)

DOWNWARD DRIFT

Lower socioeconomic groups have higher rates of schizophrenia. This may be due to the **downward drift hypothesis**, which postulates that people suffering from schizophrenia are unable to function well in society and hence end up in lower socioeconomic groups. Many homeless people in urban areas suffer from schizophrenia.

PATHOPHYSIOLOGY OF SCHIZOPHRENIA: THE DOPAMINE HYPOTHESIS

Though the exact cause of schizophrenia is not known, it appears to be partly related to increased dopamine activity in certain neuronal tracts. Evidence to support this hypothesis is that most antipsychotics successful in treating schizophrenia are dopamine receptor antagonists. In addition, cocaine and amphetamines increase dopamine activity and can cause schizophrenia-like symptoms.

KEY FACT

Schizophrenia is found in lower socioeconomic groups likely due to "downward drift" (many patients have difficulty in holding good jobs, so they tend to drift downward socioeconomically).

Theorized Dopamine Pathways Affected in Schizophrenia
- *Prefrontal cortical:* Inadequate dopaminergic activity; responsible for negative symptoms.
- *Mesolimbic:* Excessive dopaminergic activity; responsible for positive symptoms.

Other Important Dopamine Pathways Affected by Antipsychotics
- *Tuberoinfundibular:* Blocked by antipsychotics, causing hyperprolactinemia, which may lead to gynecomastia, galactorrhea, sexual dysfunction, and menstrual irregularities.
- *Nigrostriatal:* Blocked by antipsychotics, causing Parkinsonism/extrapyramidal side effects such as tremor, rigidity, slurred speech, akathisia, dystonia, and other abnormal movements.

OTHER NEUROTRANSMITTER ABNORMALITIES IMPLICATED IN SCHIZOPHRENIA

- **Elevated serotonin:** Some of the second-generation (atypical) antipsychotics (e.g., risperidone and clozapine) antagonize serotonin and weakly antagonize dopamine.
- **Elevated norepinephrine:** Long-term use of antipsychotics has been shown to decrease activity of noradrenergic neurons.
- Low **gamma-aminobutyric acid (GABA):** There is lower expression of the enzyme necessary to create GABA in the hippocampus of schizophrenic patients.
- Low **levels of glutamate receptors:** Schizophrenic patients have fewer NMDA receptors; this corresponds to the psychotic symptoms observed with NMDA antagonists like ketamine.

PROGNOSTIC FACTORS

Even with medication, 40–60% of patients remain significantly impaired after their diagnosis, while only 20–30% function fairly well in society. About 20% of patients with schizophrenia attempt suicide and many more experience suicidal ideation. Several factors are associated with a better or worse prognosis:

Associated with Better Prognosis
- Later onset.
- Good social support.
- Positive symptoms.
- Mood symptoms.
- Acute onset.
- Female gender.
- Few relapses.
- Good premorbid functioning.

Associated with Worse Prognosis
- Early onset.
- Poor social support.
- Negative symptoms.
- Family history.
- Gradual onset.

KEY FACT

Akathisia is an unpleasant, subjective sense of restlessness and need to move, often manifested by the inability to sit still.

KEY FACT

The lifetime prevalence of schizophrenia is 0.3–0.7%.

KEY FACT

Schizophrenia has a large genetic component. If one identical twin has schizophrenia, the risk of the other identical twin having schizophrenia is 50%. A biological child of a schizophrenic person has a higher chance of developing schizophrenia, even if adopted into a family without schizophrenia.

KEY FACT

Computed tomography (CT) and magnetic resonance imaging (MRI) scans of patients with schizophrenia may show enlargement of the ventricles, diffuse cortical atrophy, and reduced brain volume.

KEY FACT

Schizophrenia often involves neologisms. A neologism is a newly coined word or expression that has meaning only to the person who uses it.

- Male gender.
- Many relapses.
- Poor premorbid functioning (social isolation, etc.).
- Comorbid substance use.

TREATMENT

A multimodal approach is the most effective, and therapy must be tailored to the needs of the specific patient. **Pharmacologic** treatment consists primarily of antipsychotic medications. (For more detail, see Chapter 18, "Psychopharmacology.")

- **First-generation (or typical) antipsychotic medications** (e.g., *chlorpromazine, fluphenazine, haloperidol, perphenazine*):
    - Primarily dopamine (mostly D2) antagonists.
    - Treat positive symptoms with minimal impact on negative symptoms.
    - Side effects include extrapyramidal symptoms, neuroleptic malignant syndrome, and tardive dyskinesia (see below).
- **Second-generation (or atypical) antipsychotic medications** (e.g., *aripiprazole, asenapine, clozapine, iloperidone, lurasidone, olanzapine, quetiapine, risperidone, ziprasidone*):
    - These antagonize serotonin receptors (5-HT2) as well as dopamine (D4>D2) receptors.
    - Research has not shown a significant difference between first- and second-generation antipsychotics in efficacy. The selection requires the weighing of benefits and risks in individual clinical cases.
    - Lower incidence of extrapyramidal side effects, but higher risk of metabolic syndrome.
    - Medications should be taken for at least 4 weeks before efficacy is determined.
    - Clozapine is reserved for patients who have failed multiple antipsychotic trials due to its risk of agranulocytosis.

Behavioral therapy attempts to improve patients' ability to function in society. Patients are helped through a variety of methods to improve their social skills, become self-sufficient, and minimize disruptive behaviors. **Family therapy** and **group therapy** are also useful adjuncts.

Important Side Effects and Sequelae of Antipsychotic Medications

Side effects of antipsychotic medications include:

1. Extrapyramidal symptoms (especially with the use of high-potency first-generation antipsychotics):
    - Dystonia (spasms) of face, neck, and tongue.
    - Parkinsonism (resting tremor, rigidity, bradykinesia).
    - Akathisia (feeling of restlessness).

   Treatment: Anticholinergics (benztropine, diphenhydramine), benzodiazepines/beta-blockers (specifically for akathisia).
2. Anticholinergic symptoms (especially low-potency first-generation antipsychotics and atypical antipsychotics): Dry mouth, constipation, blurred vision, hyperthermia.

   Treatment: As per symptom (eye drops, stool softeners, etc.).
3. Metabolic syndrome (second-generation antipsychotics): A constellation of conditions—**elevated** blood pressure, **elevated** blood sugar levels, excess body fat around the waist, abnormal cholesterol levels—that occur

WARDS TIP

First-generation antipsychotic medications are referred to as typical or conventional antipsychotics (often called neuroleptics). Second-generation antipsychotic medications are referred to as atypical antipsychotics.

WARDS TIP

Patients who are treated with *first-generation* (typical) antipsychotic medication need to be closely monitored for extrapyramidal symptoms, such as acute dystonia and tardive dyskinesia.

WARDS TIP

Schizophrenic patients who are treated with *second-generation* (atypical) antipsychotic medications need a careful medical evaluation for metabolic syndrome. This includes checking weight, body mass index (BMI), fasting blood glucose or HbA1c, lipid assessment, and blood pressure.

KEY FACT

High-potency antipsychotics (such as haloperidol and fluphenazine) have a higher incidence of extrapyramidal side effects, while *low-potency* antipsychotics (such as chlorpromazine) have primarily anticholinergic and antiadrenergic side effects.

together, **increasing** the risk for cardiovascular disease, stroke, and type 2 diabetes.
Treatment: Consider switching to a first-generation antipsychotic or a more "weight-neutral" second-generation antipsychotic such as aripiprazole or ziprasidone. Consider metformin if the patient is not already on it. Monitor lipids and blood glucose measurements. Refer the patient to primary care for appropriate treatment of hyperlipidemia, diabetes, etc. Encourage appropriate diet, exercise, and smoking cessation.

4. Tardive dyskinesia (more likely with first-generation antipsychotics): Choreoathetoid movements, usually seen in the face, tongue, and head.
Treatment: Discontinue or reduce the medication and consider substituting an atypical antispsychotic (if appropriate). VMAT-2 inhibitors such as valbenzazine, benzodiazepines, Botox, and vitamin E may be used. The movements may persist despite withdrawal of the drug. Although less common, atypical antipsychotics can also cause tardive dyskinesia.

5. Neuroleptic malignant syndrome (NMS) (typically high-potency first-generation antipsychotics):
   - Change in mental status, autonomic instability (high fever, labile blood pressure, tachycardia, tachypnea, diaphoresis), "lead pipe" rigidity, elevated creatine kinase (CK) levels, leukocytosis, and metabolic acidosis. Reflexes are decreased.
   - NMS is a **medical emergency** that requires prompt withdrawal of all antipsychotic medications and immediate medical assessment and treatment.
   - May be observed in any patient being treated with any antipsychotic (including second generation) medications at any time, but is more frequently associated with the initiation of treatment and at higher IV/IM dosing of high-potency neuroleptics.
   - Patients with a history of prior neuroleptic malignant syndrome are at increased risk of recurrent episodes when retrialed with antipsychotic agents.

6. Prolonged QTc interval and other electrocardiogram changes, hyperprolactinemia (gynecomastia, galactorrhea, amenorrhea, diminished libido, and impotence), hematologic effects (agranulocytosis may occur with *clozapine*, requiring frequent blood draws when this medication is used), ophthalmologic conditions (*thioridazine* may cause irreversible retinal pigmentation at high doses; deposits in lens and cornea may occur with *chlorpromazine*), dermatologic conditions (such as rashes and photosensitivity).

Schizophreniform Disorder

Diagnosis and DSM-5 Criteria

The diagnosis of schizophreniform disorder is made using the same DSM-5 criteria as schizophrenia. The only difference is that in schizophreniform disorder the symptoms have lasted between 1 and 6 months, whereas in schizophrenia the symptoms must be present for >6 months.

Prognosis

One-third of patients recover completely; two-thirds progress to schizoaffective disorder or schizophrenia.

Tardive dyskinesia occurs most often in older women after at least 6 months of medication. A small percentage of patients will experience spontaneous remission, so discontinuation of the agent should be considered if clinically appropriate.

The cumulative risk of developing tardive dyskinesia from antipsychotics (particularly first generation) is 5% per year.

Clozapine is typically considered for treating schizophrenia when a patient fails both typical and other atypical antipsychotics. It is a very effective medication, but as it can rarely cause agranulocytosis, patients must be monitored (WBC and absolute neutrophil counts) regularly.

If a schizophrenia presentation has not been present for 6 months, think *schizophreniform disorder.*

Treatment

Hospitalization (if necessary), 6-month course of antipsychotics, and supportive psychotherapy.

Schizoaffective Disorder

Diagnosis and DSM-5 Criteria

The diagnosis of schizoaffective disorder is made in patients who:

- Meet criteria for either a major depressive or manic episode during which psychotic symptoms consistent with schizophrenia are also met.
- Delusions or hallucinations for 2 weeks in the absence of mood disorder symptoms (this criterion is necessary to differentiate schizoaffective disorder from a mood disorder with psychotic features).
- Mood symptoms present for a majority of the psychotic illness.
- Symptoms not due to the effects of a substance (drug or medication) or another medical condition.

Prognosis

Worse with poor premorbid adjustment, slow onset, early onset, predominance of psychotic symptoms, long course, and family history of schizophrenia.

Treatment

- Hospitalization (if necessary) and supportive psychotherapy.
- Medical therapy: Antipsychotics (second-generation medications may target both psychotic and mood symptoms); mood stabilizers, antidepressants, or electroconvulsive therapy (ECT) may be indicated for treatment of mood symptoms.

 KEY FACT

Patients with borderline personality disorder may have transient, stress-related psychotic experiences. These are considered part of their underlying personality disorder and are not diagnosed as a brief psychotic disorder.

Brief Psychotic Disorder

Diagnosis and DSM-5 Criteria

Patient with psychotic symptoms as in schizophrenia; however, the symptoms last from 1 day to 1 month, and there must be eventual full return to premorbid level of functioning. Symptoms must not be due to the effects of a substance (drug or medication) or another medical condition. This is a rare diagnosis, much less common than schizophrenia. It may be seen in reaction to extreme stress such as bereavement and sexual assault.

Prognosis

High rates of relapse, but almost all completely recover.

Treatment

Brief hospitalization (usually required for workup, safety, and stabilization), supportive therapy, course of antipsychotics for psychosis, and/or benzodiazepines for agitation.

Delusional Disorder

Delusional disorder occurs more often in middle-aged or older patients (after age 40). Immigrants, the hearing impaired, and those with a family history of schizophrenia are at increased risk.

Diagnosis and DSM-5 Criteria

To be diagnosed with delusional disorder, the following criteria must be met:

- One or more delusions for at least 1 month.
- Does not meet criteria for schizophrenia.
- Functioning in life not significantly impaired, and behavior not obviously bizarre.
- While delusions may be present in both delusional disorder and schizophrenia, there are important differences (see Table 3-1).

Types of Delusions

Patients are further categorized based on the types of delusions they experience:

- **Erotomanic type:** Delusion that another person is in love with the individual.
- **Grandiose type:** Delusions of having great talent.
- **Somatic type:** Physical delusions.
- **Persecutory type:** Delusions of being persecuted.
- **Jealous type:** Delusions of unfaithfulness.
- **Mixed type:** More than one of the above.
- **Unspecified type:** Not a specific type as described above.

Prognosis

Better than schizophrenia with treatment:

- >50%: Full recovery.
- >20%: Symptoms.
- <20%: No change.

Treatment

Difficult to treat, especially given the lack of insight and impairment. Antipsychotic medications are recommended despite somewhat limited evidence. Supportive therapy is often helpful.

TABLE 3-1. Schizophrenia versus Delusional Disorder

Schizophrenia	Delusional Disorder

■ Bizarre or nonbizarre delusions
■ Daily functioning significantly impaired
■ Must have two or more of the following:
  ■ Delusions
  ■ Hallucinations
  ■ Disorganized speech
  ■ Disorganized behavior
  ■ Negative symptoms
	■ Usually nonbizarre delusions
	■ Daily functioning not significantly impaired
	■ Does not meet the criteria for schizophrenia, as described in the left column

Culture-Specific Psychoses

The following are examples of psychotic disorders seen within certain cultures:

	Psychotic Manifestation	Culture
Koro	Intense anxiety that the penis will recede into the body, possibly leading to death.	Southeast Asia (e.g., Singapore)
Amok	Sudden unprovoked outbursts of violence, often followed by suicide.	Malaysia
Brain fag	Headache, fatigue, eye pain, cognitive difficulties, and other somatic disturbances in male students.	Africa

Comparing Time Courses and Prognoses of Psychotic Disorders

Time Course

- <1 month—brief psychotic disorder.
- 1–6 months—schizophreniform disorder.
- >6 months—schizophrenia.

Prognosis from Best to Worst

Mood disorder with psychotic features > schizoaffective disorder > schizophreniform disorder > schizophrenia.

> **QUICK AND EASY DISTINGUISHING FEATURES**
>
> - **Schizophrenia:** Lifelong psychotic disorder.
> - **Schizophreniform:** Schizophrenia for >1 and <6 months.
> - **Schizoaffective:** Distinct mood episodes with psychosis persisting between mood episodes.
> - **Schizotypal** (personality disorder): Paranoid, odd or magical beliefs, eccentric, lack of friends, social anxiety. Criteria for overt psychosis are not met.
> - **Schizoid** (personality disorder): Solitary activities, lack of enjoyment from social interactions, no psychosis.

KEY FACT

SchizophreniFORM = the FORMation of a schizophrenic, but not quite there (i.e., <6 months).

NOTES

CHAPTER 4

MOOD DISORDERS

Concepts in Mood Disorders	36
Mood Disorders versus Mood Episodes	36
Mood Episodes	36
Major Depressive Episode (MDE)	36
Manic Episode	36
Hypomanic Episode	37
Differences between Manic and Hypomanic Episodes	37
Mixed Features	37
Mood Disorders	37
Differential Diagnosis of Mood Disorders Due to Other Medical Conditions	37
Substance/Medication-Induced Mood Disorders	38
Major Depressive Disorder (MDD)	39
Specifiers for Depressive Disorders	41
Bereavement	42
Bipolar I Disorder	42
Bipolar II Disorder	43
Specifiers for Bipolar Disorders	44
Persistent Depressive Disorder (Dysthymia)	44
Cyclothymic Disorder	45
Premenstrual Dysphoric Disorder	46
Disruptive Mood Dysregulation Disorder (DMDD)	46
Other Disorders of Mood in DSM-5	47

Concepts in Mood Disorders

A **mood** is a description of one's internal emotional state. Both external and internal stimuli can trigger moods, which may be labeled as sad, happy, angry, irritable, and so on. It is normal to have a wide range of moods and to have a sense of control over one's moods.

Patients with mood *disorders* (also called affective disorders) experience an abnormal range of moods and lose some level of control over them. Distress may be caused by the severity of their moods and the resulting impairment in social and occupational functioning.

WARDS TIP

Major depressive episodes can be present in major depressive disorder, persistent depressive disorder (dysthymia), bipolar I/II disorder, and schizoaffective disorder.

Mood Disorders versus Mood Episodes

- **Mood episodes** are distinct periods of time in which some abnormal mood is present. They include depression, mania, and hypomania.
- **Mood disorders** are defined by their patterns of mood episodes. They include major depressive disorder (MDD), bipolar I disorder, bipolar II disorder, persistent depressive disorder, and cyclothymic disorder. Some may have psychotic features (delusions or hallucinations).

WARDS TIP

When patients have delusions and hallucinations due to underlying mood disorders, they are usually mood congruent. For example, depression causes psychotic themes of paranoia and worthlessness, and mania causes psychotic themes of grandiosity and invincibility.

Mood Episodes

MAJOR DEPRESSIVE EPISODE (MDE)

Must have at least five of the following symptoms (must include either number 1 or 2) for at least a 2-week period:

1. Depressed mood most of the time.
2. Anhedonia (loss of interest in pleasurable activities).
3. Change in appetite or weight (↑ or ↓).
4. Feelings of worthlessness or excessive guilt.
5. Insomnia or hypersomnia.
6. Diminished concentration.
7. Psychomotor agitation or retardation (i.e., restlessness or slowness).
8. Fatigue or loss of energy.
9. Recurrent thoughts of death or suicide.

Symptoms must not be attributable to the effects of a substance (drug or medication) or another medical condition, and they must cause clinically significant distress or social/occupational impairment.

KEY FACT

Symptoms of major depression—
SIG E. CAPS (Prescribe Energy Capsules)
Sleep
Interest
Guilt
Energy
Concentration
Appetite
Psychomotor activity
Suicidal ideation

MANIC EPISODE

A distinct period of abnormally and persistently elevated, expansive, or irritable mood, and abnormally and persistently increased goal-directed activity or energy, lasting at least 1 week (or any duration if hospitalization is necessary), and including at least three of the following (four if the mood is only irritable):

1. Distractibility.
2. Inflated self-esteem or grandiosity.
3. ↑ in goal-directed activity (socially, at work, or sexually) or psychomotor agitation.

4. ↓ need for sleep.
5. Flight of ideas or racing thoughts.
6. More talkative than usual or *pressured speech* (rapid and uninterruptible).
7. Excessive involvement in pleasurable activities that have a high risk of negative consequences (e.g., shopping sprees, sexual indiscretions).

Symptoms must not be attributable to the effects of a substance (drug or medication) or another medical condition, and they must cause clinically significant distress or social/occupational impairment. Greater than 50% of patients with manic episodes have psychotic symptoms.

HYPOMANIC EPISODE

A hypomanic episode is a distinct period of abnormally and persistently elevated, expansive, or irritable mood, and abnormally and persistently increased goal-directed activity or energy, lasting at least 4 consecutive days, that includes at least three of the symptoms listed for the manic episode criteria (four if mood is only irritable). There are significant differences between mania and hypomania (see below).

DIFFERENCES BETWEEN MANIC AND HYPOMANIC EPISODES

Mania	Hypomania
Lasts at least 7 days	Lasts at least 4 days
Causes severe impairment in social or occupational functioning	No marked impairment in social or occupational functioning
May necessitate hospitalization to prevent harm to self or others	Does not require hospitalization
May have psychotic features	No psychotic features

MIXED FEATURES

Criteria are met for a manic or hypomanic episode and at least three symptoms of a major depressive episode are present for the majority of the time. These criteria must be present nearly every day for at least 1 week.

Mood Disorders

Mood disorders often have chronic courses that are marked by relapses *with relatively normal functioning between episodes*. Like most psychiatric diagnoses, mood episodes may be caused by another medical condition or drug (prescribed or illicit). Therefore, always investigate medical or substance-induced causes (see below) before making a primary psychiatric diagnosis.

DIFFERENTIAL DIAGNOSIS OF MOOD DISORDERS DUE TO OTHER MEDICAL CONDITIONS

Medical Causes of a Depressive Episode

Cerebrovascular disease (stroke, myocardial infarction)
Endocrinopathies (diabetes mellitus, Cushing syndrome, Addison disease,

Medical Causes of a Manic Episode

Metabolic (hyperthyroidism)
Neurological disorders (temporal lobe seizures, multiple sclerosis)

KEY FACT

Symptoms of mania—
DIG FAST
Distractibility
Insomnia/Impulsive behavior
Grandiosity
Flight of ideas/Racing thoughts
Activity/Agitation
Speech (pressured)
Thoughtlessness

WARDS TIP

A manic episode is a psychiatric emergency; severely impaired judgment can make a patient dangerous to self and others.

WARDS TIP

Irritability is often the predominant mood state in mood disorders with mixed features. Patients with mixed features have a poorer response to lithium. Anticonvulsants such as valproic acid may be more helpful.

KEY FACT

Stroke patients are at a significant risk for developing depression, and this is associated with a poorer outcome overall.

KEY FACT

Depression is common in patients with pancreatic cancer.

hypoglycemia, hyper/hypothyroidism, hyper/hypocalcemia)
Parkinson disease
Viral illnesses (e.g., mononucleosis)
Carcinoid syndrome
Cancer (especially lymphoma and pancreatic carcinoma)
Collagen vascular disease (e.g., systemic lupus erythematosus)

Neoplasms
HIV infection

SUBSTANCE/MEDICATION-INDUCED MOOD DISORDERS

Substance/Medication-Induced Depressive Disorder

EtOH
Antihypertensives
Barbiturates
Corticosteroids
Levodopa
Sedative-hypnotics
Anticonvulsants
Antipsychotics
Diuretics
Sulfonamides
Withdrawal from stimulants (e.g., cocaine, amphetamines)

Substance/Medication-Induced Bipolar Disorder

Antidepressants
Sympathomimetics
Dopamine
Corticosteroids
Levodopa
Bronchodilators
Cocaine
Amphetamines

> Ms. Cruz is a 28-year-old sales clerk who arrives at your outpatient clinic complaining of sadness after her boyfriend of 6 months ended their relationship 1 month ago. She describes a history of failed romantic relationships, and says, "I don't do well with breakups." Ms. Cruz reports that, although she has no prior psychiatric treatment, she was urged by her employer to seek therapy. Ms. Cruz has arrived late to work on several occasions because of oversleeping. She also has difficulty in getting out of bed stating, "It's difficult to walk; it's like my legs weigh a ton." She feels fatigued during the day despite spending over 12 hours in bed, and is concerned that she might be suffering from a serious medical condition. She denies any significant changes in appetite or weight since these symptoms began.
>
> Ms. Cruz reports that, although she has not missed workdays, she has difficulty concentrating and has become tearful in front of clients while worrying about not finding a significant other. She feels tremendous guilt over "not being good enough to get married," and says that her close friends are concerned because she has been spending her weekends in bed and not answering their calls. Although during your evaluation Ms. Cruz appears tearful, she brightens up when talking about her newborn nephew and her plans to visit a college friend next summer. Ms. Cruz denies suicidal ideation.
>
> ### What is Ms. Cruz's diagnosis?
>
> Ms. Cruz's diagnosis is major depressive disorder with atypical features. She complains of sadness, fatigue, poor concentration, hypersomnia,

feelings of guilt, anhedonia, and impairment in her social and occupational functioning. The atypical features specifier is given in this case as she exhibited mood reactivity (mood brightens in response to positive events) when talking about her nephew and visiting her friend, and complained of a heavy feeling in her legs (leaden paralysis) and hypersomnia. It is also important to explore Ms. Cruz's history of "not doing well with breakups," as this could be indicative of a long pattern of interpersonal rejection sensitivity. Although it is common for patients who suffer from atypical depression to report an ↑ in appetite, Ms. Cruz exhibits enough symptoms to fulfill atypical features criteria. Adjustment disorder should also be considered in the differential diagnosis.

What would be your pharmacological recommendation?

Ms. Cruz should be treated with an antidepressant medication. While MAOIs such as phenelzine had traditionally been superior to TCAs in the treatment of MDD with atypical features, SSRIs would be the first-line treatment. The combination of pharmacotherapy and psychotherapy has been shown to be more effective for treating mild-to-moderate MDD than either treatment alone.

MAJOR DEPRESSIVE DISORDER (MDD)

Major depressive disorder (MDD) is marked by episodes of depressed mood associated with loss of interest in daily activities. Patients may not acknowledge their depressed mood or may express vague, somatic complaints (fatigue, headache, abdominal pain, muscle tension, etc.).

Diagnosis and DSM-5 Criteria
- At least one major depressive episode (see above).
- No history of manic or hypomanic episode.

Epidemiology
- Lifetime prevalence: 12% worldwide.
- Onset at any age, but the age of onset peaks in the 20s.
- 1.5–2 times as prevalent in women than men during reproductive years.
- No ethnic or socioeconomic differences.
- Lifetime prevalence in the elderly: <10%.
- Depression can ↑ mortality for patients with other comorbidities such as diabetes, stroke, and cardiovascular disease.

Sleep Problems Associated with MDD
- Multiple awakenings.
- Initial and terminal insomnia (hard to fall asleep and early morning awakenings).
- Hypersomnia (excessive sleepiness) is less common.
- Rapid eye movement (REM) sleep shifted earlier in the night and for a greater duration, with reduced stages 3 and 4 (slow wave) sleep.

Etiology

The precise cause of depression is unknown, but MDD is believed to be a heterogeneous disease, with biological, genetic, environmental, and psychosocial factors contributing.

KEY FACT

Anhedonia is the inability to experience pleasure, which is a common finding in depression.

KEY FACT

Major depressive disorder is the most common disorder among those who commit suicide.

WARDS TIP

The two most common types of sleep disturbances associated with MDD are difficulty falling asleep and early morning awakenings.

- MDD is likely caused by neurotransmitter abnormalities in the brain. Evidence for this is the following: antidepressants exert their therapeutic effect by increasing catecholamines; ↓ cerebrospinal fluid (CSF) levels of 5-hydroxyindolacetic acid (5-HIAA), the main metabolite of serotonin, have been found in depressed patients with impulsive and suicidal behavior.
- Increased sensitivity of beta-adrenergic receptors in the brain has also been postulated in the pathogenesis of MDD.
- **High cortisol:** Hyperactivity of hypothalamic-pituitary-adrenal axis, as shown by failure to suppress cortisol levels in the dexamethasone suppression test.
- **Abnormal thyroid axis:** Thyroid disorders are associated with depressive symptoms.
- Gamma-aminobutyric acid (GABA), glutamate, and endogenous opiates may additionally have a role.
- **Psychosocial/life events:** Multiple adverse childhood experiences are a risk factor for later developing MDD.
- **Genetics:** First-degree relatives are two to four times more likely to have MDD. Concordance rate for monozygotic twins is <40%, and 10–20% for dizygotic twins.

Course and Prognosis

- Untreated, depressive episodes are self-limiting but last from 6 to 12 months. Generally, episodes occur more frequently as the disorder progresses. The risk of a subsequent major depressive episode is 50–60% within the first 2 years after the first episode. Up to 15% of patients with MDD eventually commit suicide.
- Approximately 60–70% of patients show a significant response to antidepressants. Combined treatment with both an antidepressant and psychotherapy produce a significantly ↑ response for MDD.

Treatment

Hospitalization

- Indicated if the patient is at risk for suicide, homicide, or is unable to care for him/herself.

Pharmacotherapy

- **Antidepressant medications:**
  - *Selective serotonin reuptake inhibitors (SSRIs):* Inhibit the reuptake of serotonin, thus increasing the amount of serotonin in the brain. Safer and better tolerated than other classes of antidepressants; side effects are mild but include headache, *gastrointestinal disturbance, sexual dysfunction*, and rebound anxiety. Examples are fluoxetine (Prozac®) escitalopram (Lexapro®) and sertraline (Zoloft®).
  - *Serotonin-norepinephrine reuptake inhibitors (SNRIs):* Inhibit the reuptake of both serotonin and norepinephrine, thus increasing the level of both neurotransmitters in the brain. Includes venlafaxine (Effexor®) and duloxetine (Cymbalta®).
  - *Novel agents:* Other agents commonly used to treat depression include the α2-adrenergic receptor antagonist mirtazapine (Remeron®), and the dopamine-norepinephrine reuptake inhibitor bupropion (Wellbutrin®).
  - *Tricyclic antidepressants (TCAs):* Most lethal in overdose due to cardiac arrhythmias; side effects include sedation, weight gain, orthostatic hypotension, and anticholinergic effects. Can aggravate prolonged QTc syndrome.

KEY FACT

The Hamilton Depression Rating Scale measures the severity of depression and is used in research to assess the effectiveness of therapies. PHQ-9 is a depression screening form often used in the primary care setting.

KEY FACT

Loss of a parent before age 11 is associated with the later development of major depression.

KEY FACT

Most adults with depression do not see a mental health professional, but they often present to a primary care physician for other reasons.

KEY FACT

Only half of patients with MDD receive treatment.

- *Monoamine oxidase inhibitors (MAOIs):* Older medications occasionally used for refractory depression; risk of *hypertensive crisis* when used with sympathomimetics or ingestion of tyramine-rich foods, such as wine, beer, aged cheeses, liver, and smoked meats (tyramine is an intermediate in the conversion of tyrosine to norepinephrine); risk of *serotonin syndrome* when used in combination with SSRIs. Most common side effect is orthostatic hypotension.
- **Adjunct medications:**
  - Atypical (second-generation) antipsychotics along with antidepressants are first-line treatment in patients with MDD with psychotic features. In addition, they may also be prescribed in patients with treatment resistant/refractory MDD without psychotic features.
  - Triiodothyronine (T3), levothyroxine (T4), and lithium have demonstrated some benefit when augmenting antidepressants in treatment refractory MDD.
  - While stimulants (such as methylphenidate) may be used in certain patients (e.g., geriatric and terminally ill patients), the efficacy is limited and trials are small.

Psychotherapy

- Cognitive-behavioral therapy (CBT), interpersonal psychotherapy, supportive therapy, psychodynamic psychotherapy, problem-solving therapy, and family/couples therapy have all demonstrated benefit in treating MDD.
  - Among the major kinds of psychotherapy, there is no compelling evidence that one is superior to the rest. The choice is usually based on availability and patient preference.
  - CBT and interpersonal psychotherapy are often selected as initial treatment because they have been the most widely studied.
- May be used alone or in conjunction with pharmacotherapy.
- Early dropout is common (as with pharmacotherapy). It is important to track patient adherence over time.

Electroconvulsive Therapy (ECT)

- Indicated if the patient is unresponsive to pharmacotherapy, if patient cannot tolerate pharmacotherapy (pregnancy, etc.), or if rapid reduction of symptoms is desired (e.g., immediate suicide risk, refusal to eat/drink, catatonia).
- ECT is extremely safe (primary risk is from anesthesia) and may be used alone or in combination with pharmacotherapy.
- ECT is often performed by premedication with atropine, followed by general anesthesia (usually with methohexital) and administration of a muscle relaxant (typically succinylcholine). A generalized seizure is then induced by passing a current of electricity across the brain (either bilateral or unilateral); the seizure should last between 30 and 60 seconds, and no longer than 90 seconds.
- 6–12 treatments are administered over a 2- to 3-week period, but significant improvement is sometimes noted after the first several treatments.
- Retrograde and anterograde amnesia are common side effects, which usually resolve within 6 months.
- Other common but transient side effects: headache, nausea, muscle soreness.

SPECIFIERS FOR DEPRESSIVE DISORDERS

- **Melancholic features:** Present in approximately 25–30% of patients with a MDE and more likely in severely ill inpatients, including those with psychotic features. Characterized by *anhedonia*, early morning awakenings,

WARDS TIP

MAOIs were considered particularly useful in the treatment of "atypical" depression; however, SSRIs remain first-line treatment for major depressive episodes with atypical features.

KEY FACT

All antidepressant medications are equally effective but differ in side-effect profiles. Medications usually take 4–6 weeks to fully work.

WARDS TIP

Serotonin syndrome is marked by autonomic instability, hyperthermia, hyperreflexia (including myoclonus), and seizures. Coma or death may result.

WARDS TIP

Adjunctive treatment is usually performed after multiple first-line treatment failures.

KEY FACT

The postpartum period conveys an elevated risk of depression in women.

depression worse in the morning, psychomotor disturbance, excessive guilt, and anorexia. For example, you may diagnose major depressive disorder with melancholic features.
- **Atypical features:** Characterized by hypersomnia, hyperphagia, reactive mood, leaden paralysis, and hypersensitivity to interpersonal rejection.
- **Mixed features:** Manic/hypomanic symptoms present during the majority of days during a MDE: elevated mood, grandiosity, talkativeness/pressured speech, flight of ideas/racing thoughts, increased energy/goal-directed activity, excessive involvement in dangerous activities, and decreased need for sleep.
- **Catatonia:** Features include catalepsy (immobility), purposeless motor activity, extreme negativism or mutism, bizarre postures, and echolalia. Especially responsive to ECT. (May also be applied to bipolar disorder.)
- **Psychotic features:** Characterized by the presence of delusions and/or hallucinations. Present in 24–53% of older, hospitalized patients with MDD.
- **Anxious distress:** Defined by feeling keyed up/tense, restless, difficulty concentrating, fears of something bad happening, and feelings of loss of control.
- **Peripartum onset:** Onset of MDD symptoms occurs during pregnancy or 4 weeks following delivery.
- **Seasonal pattern:** Temporal relationship between the onset of a MDE and particular time of the year (most commonly the winter but may occur in any season). Patients with fall-onset SAD (seasonal affective disorder or "winter depression") often respond to light therapy.

WARDS TIP

Triad for seasonal affective disorder:
- Irritability
- Carbohydrate craving
- Hypersomnia

WARDS TIP

Major depression with psychotic features is best treated with a combination of an antidepressant **and** antipsychotic, **or** ECT.

KEY FACT

Bereavement is NOT a DSM-5 diagnosis—if a patient meets criteria for major depression following the loss of a loved one, the diagnosis is major depression.

BEREAVEMENT

Bereavement, also known as simple grief, is a reaction to a major loss, usually of a loved one, and it is not a mental illness. While symptoms are usually self-limited and only last for several months, if an individual meets criteria for a depressive episode, he/she would be diagnosed with MDD. Normal bereavement should not include gross psychotic symptoms, disorganization, or active suicidality.

BIPOLAR I DISORDER

Bipolar I disorder involves episodes of mania and of major depression; however, episodes of major depression are *not* required for the diagnosis. It is also known as **manic-depression**.

Diagnosis and DSM-5 Criteria

The only requirement for this diagnosis is the occurrence of a **manic episode** (5% of patients experience only manic episodes). Between manic episodes, there may be interspersed euthymia, major depressive episodes, or hypomanic episodes, but none of these are required for the diagnosis.

Epidemiology

- Lifetime prevalence: 1–2%.
- Women and men are equally affected.
- No ethnic differences seen; however, high-income countries have twice the rate of low-income countries (1.4% versus 0.7%).
- Onset usually before age 30, mean age of first mood episode is 18.
- Frequently misdiagnosed and thereby inappropriately or inadequately treated.

Etiology

- Biological, environmental, psychosocial, and genetic factors are all important.
- First-degree relatives of patients with bipolar disorder are 10 times more likely to develop the illness.
- Concordance rates for monozygotic twins are 40–70%, and rates for dizygotic twins range from 5% to 25%.
- Bipolar I has the highest genetic link of all major psychiatric disorders.

Course and Prognosis

- Untreated manic episodes generally last several months.
- The course is usually chronic with relapses; as the disease progresses, episodes may occur more frequently.
- Ninety percent of individuals after one manic episode will have a repeat mood episode within 5 years.
- Bipolar disorder has a poorer prognosis than MDD.
- Maintenance treatment with mood stabilizing medications between episodes helps to ↓ the risk of relapse.
- 25 to 50% of people with bipolar disorder attempt suicide, and 10–15% die by suicide.

Treatment

- **Pharmacotherapy:**
    - Lithium is a mood stabilizer; 50–70% treated with lithium show partial reduction of mania. Long-term use **reduces suicide risk**. Acute overdose can be fatal due to its low therapeutic index.
    - The anticonvulsants carbamazepine and valproic acid are also mood stabilizers. They are particularly useful for rapid cycling bipolar disorder and those with mixed features.
    - Atypical antipsychotics (e.g., risperidone, olanzapine, quetiapine, ziprasidone) are effective as both monotherapy and adjunct therapy for acute mania. In fact, many patients (especially with severe mania and/or with psychotic features) are treated with a combination of a mood stabilizer and antipsychotic; studies have shown a greater and faster response with combination therapy.
    - Antidepressants are discouraged as monotherapy due to concerns of activating mania or hypomania. They are occasionally used to treat depressive episodes when patients concurrently take mood stabilizers.
- **Psychotherapy:** Supportive psychotherapy, family therapy, group therapy (may prolong remission once the acute manic episode has been controlled).
- **ECT:**
    - Works well in treatment of manic episodes.
    - Some patients require more treatments (up to 20) than for depression.
    - Especially effective for refractory or life-threatening acute mania or depression.

KEY FACT

Treatment for bipolar disorder includes lithium, valproic acid, and carbamazepine (for rapid cyclers), or second-generation antipsychotics. Lithium remains the gold standard, particularly due to demonstrated reduction in suicide risk.

WARDS TIP

Side effects of lithium include:
- Weight gain
- Tremor
- Gastrointestinal disturbances
- Fatigue
- Cardiac arrhythmias
- Seizures
- Goiter/hypothyroidism
- Leukocytosis (benign)
- Coma (in toxic doses)
- Polyuria (nephrogenic diabetes insipidus)
- Polydipsia
- Alopecia
- Metallic taste

KEY FACT

ECT is the best treatment for a pregnant woman who is having a manic episode. It provides a good alternative to antipsychotics and can be used with relative safety in all trimesters.

BIPOLAR II DISORDER

Alternatively thought of as **recurrent major depressive episodes with hypomania.**

Diagnosis and DSM-5 Criteria

History of one or more major depressive episodes and at least one **hypomanic** episode. *Remember:* If there has been a full manic episode, *even in* *the past,* or if the patient ever has a history of psychosis, then the diagnosis is bipolar I, *not* bipolar II disorder.

Epidemiology

- Prevalence is unclear, with some studies greater and others less than bipolar I.
- May be slightly more common in women.
- Onset usually before age 30.
- No ethnic differences seen.
- Frequently misdiagnosed as unipolar depression and thereby inappropriately treated.

Etiology

Same as bipolar I disorder (see above).

Course and Prognosis

Tends to be chronic, requiring long-term treatment. Likely better prognosis than bipolar I.

Treatment

Fewer studies focus on the treatment for bipolar II. Currently, treatment is the same as bipolar I disorder (see above).

SPECIFIERS FOR BIPOLAR DISORDERS

- **Anxious distress:** Defined by feeling keyed up/tense, restless, difficulty concentrating, fears of something bad happening, and feelings of loss of control.
- **Mixed features:** Depressive symptoms present during the majority of days during mania/hypomania: dysphoria/depressed mood, anhedonia, psychomotor retardation, fatigue/loss of energy, feelings of worthlessness or inappropriate guilt, thoughts of death or suicidal ideation.
- **Rapid cycling:** At least four mood episodes (manic, hypomanic, depressed) within 12 months.
- **Melancholic features** (*during depressed episode*): Characterized by *anhedonia*, early morning awakenings, depression worse in the morning, psychomotor disturbance, excessive guilt, and anorexia.
- **Atypical features** (*during depressed episode*): Characterized by hypersomnia, hyperphagia, reactive mood, leaden paralysis, and hypersensitivity to interpersonal rejection.
- **Psychotic features:** Characterized by the presence of delusions and/or hallucinations.
- **Catatonia:** Catalepsy, purposeless motor activity, extreme negativism or mutism, bizarre postures, and echolalia. Especially responsive to ECT.
- **Peripartum onset:** Onset of manic or hypomanic symptoms occurs during pregnancy or 4 weeks following delivery.
- **Seasonal pattern:** Temporal relationship between onset of mania/hypomania and particular time of the year.

PERSISTENT DEPRESSIVE DISORDER (DYSTHYMIA)

Patients with persistent depressive disorder (dysthymia) have chronic depression most of the time, and they may have discrete major depressive episodes.

KEY FACT

A patient with a history of postpartum mania has a high risk of relapse with future deliveries and should be treated with mood stabilizing agents as prophylaxis. However, some of these medications may be contraindicated in breastfeeding.

KEY FACT

Rapid cycling is defined by the occurrence of four or more mood episodes (major depressive, hypomanic, or manic) in 1 year.

WARDS TIP

Bipolar I disorder may have psychotic features (delusions or hallucinations); these can occur during major depressive *or* manic episodes. Remember to always include bipolar disorder in the differential diagnoses of a psychotic patient.

Diagnosis and DSM-5 Criteria

1. Depressed mood for the majority of time most days for at least 2 years (in children or adolescents for at least 1 year).
2. At least two of the following:
   - Poor concentration or difficulty making decisions.
   - Feelings of hopelessness.
   - Poor appetite or overeating.
   - Insomnia or hypersomnia.
   - Low energy or fatigue.
   - Low self-esteem.
3. During the 2-year period:
   - The person has not been without the above symptoms for >2 months at a time.
   - May have major depressive episode(s) or meet criteria for major depression continuously.
   - The patient must never have had a manic or hypomanic episode (this would make the diagnosis bipolar disorder or cyclothymic disorder, respectively).

Epidemiology

- Twelve-month prevalence: 2%.
- More common in women.
- Onset often in childhood, adolescence, and early adulthood.

Course and Prognosis

Early and insidious onset, with a chronic course. Depressive symptoms much less likely to resolve than in MDD.

Treatment

- Combination treatment with psychotherapy and pharmacotherapy is more efficacious than either alone.
- Cognitive therapy, interpersonal therapy, and insight-oriented psychotherapy are the most effective.
- Antidepressants found to be beneficial include SSRIs, SNRIs, novel antidepressants (e.g., bupropion, mirtazapine), TCAs, and MAOIs.

CYCLOTHYMIC DISORDER

Alternating periods of hypomania and periods with mild-to-moderate depressive symptoms.

Diagnosis and DSM-5 Criteria

- Numerous periods with hypomanic symptoms (but not a full hypomanic episode) and periods with depressive symptoms (but not full MDE) for at least 2 years.
- The person must never have been symptom free for >2 months during those 2 years.
- No history of major depressive episode, hypomania, or manic episode.

Epidemiology

- Lifetime prevalence: <1%.
- May coexist with borderline personality disorder.
- Onset usually between ages 15–25.
- Occurs equally in males and females.

WARDS TIP

Persistent **D**epressive **D**isorder (**DD**) = 2 **D**s
2 years of depression
2 listed criteria
Never asymptomatic for > 2 months

WARDS TIP

Symptoms of persistent depressive disorder (dysthymia)—two or more of: CHASES
Poor **C**oncentration or difficulty making decisions
Feelings of **H**opelessness
Poor **A**ppetite or overeating
In**S**omnia or hypersomnia
Low **E**nergy or fatigue
Low **S**elf-esteem

WARDS TIP

MDD is an episodic illness, while persistent depressive disorder is pervasive.

Course and Prognosis

Chronic course; approximately one-third of patients eventually develop bipolar I/II disorder.

Treatment

Antimanic agents (mood stabilizers or second-generation antipsychotics) as are used to treat bipolar disorder (see above).

PREMENSTRUAL DYSPHORIC DISORDER

Mood lability, irritability, dysphoria, and anxiety that occur repeatedly during the premenstrual phase of the cycle.

Diagnosis and DSM-5 Criteria

- In most menstrual cycles, at least five symptoms (below) are present in the final week before menses, improve within a few days after menses, and are minimal/absent in the week postmenses (should be confirmed by daily ratings for at least two menstrual cycles).
- At least one of the following symptoms is present: affective lability, irritability/anger, depressed mood, anxiety/tension.
- At least one of the following symptoms is present (for total of at least five symptoms when combined with above): anhedonia, problems concentrating, anergia, appetite changes/food cravings, hypersomnia/insomnia, feeling overwhelmed/out of control, physical symptoms (e.g., breast tenderness/swelling, joint/muscle pain, bloating, weight gain).
- Symptoms cause clinically significant distress or impairment in functioning.
- Symptoms are not only exacerbation of another disorder (e.g., MDD, panic disorder, persistent depressive disorder).
- Symptoms are not due to a substance (medication or drug) or another medical condition.

Epidemiology/Etiology

- Prevalence: 1.8%.
- Onset can occur at any time after menarche.
- Has been observed worldwide.
- Environmental and genetic factors contribute.

Course and Prognosis

Symptoms may worsen prior to menopause but cease after menopause.

Treatment

SSRIs are first-line treatment, either as daily therapy or luteal phase-only treatment (starting on cycle day 14 and stopping upon menses or shortly thereafter). Oral contraceptives may reduce symptoms. Gonadotropin-releasing hormone (GnRH) agonists have also been used, and, in rare, severe cases, bilateral oophorectomy with hysterectomy will resolve symptoms.

DISRUPTIVE MOOD DYSREGULATION DISORDER (DMDD)

Chronic, severe, persistent irritability occurring in childhood and adolescence.

Diagnosis and DSM-5 Criteria

- Severe recurrent verbal and/or physical outbursts out of proportion to situation.
- Outbursts ≥3 per week and inconsistent with developmental level.
- Mood between outbursts is persistently angry/irritable most of the day nearly every day, and is observed by others.
- Symptoms for at least 1 year, and no more than 3 months without symptoms.
- Symptoms in at least two settings (e.g., home, school, peers).
- Symptoms must have started before age 10, but diagnosis can be made from ages 6 to 18.
- No episodes meeting full criteria for manic/hypomanic episode lasting longer than 1 day.
- Behaviors do not occur during MDD and not better explained by another mental disorder (this disorder cannot coexist with oppositional defiant disorder, intermittent explosive disorder, or bipolar disorder).
- Symptoms not due to a substance (medication or drug) or another medical condition.

Epidemiology/Etiology

- Prevalence is unclear as this is a new diagnosis.
- 6 to 12-month prevalence rates of chronic/severe persistent irritability in children: 2–5%.
- Rates likely greater in males than females.

Course and Prognosis

- By definition, DMDD must occur prior to 10 years of age.
- Approximately 50% of those with DMDD continue to meet criteria after 1 year.
- Rates of conversion to bipolar disorder are very low.
- Very high rates of comorbidity, especially with ODD, ADHD, mood disorders, and anxiety disorders.

Treatment

- Given the new nature of this disorder, there are no consensus evidenced-based treatments. Psychotherapy, such as parent management training, for the patient and family is generally first line.
- Medications should be used to treat comorbid disorders.
- Stimulants, SSRIs, mood stabilizers, and second-generation antipsychotics have all been used to treat the primary symptoms of DMDD.

OTHER DISORDERS OF MOOD IN DSM-5

- Mood disorder due to another medical condition.
- Substance/Medication-induced mood disorder.
- Specified depressive/bipolar disorder (meets criteria for MDE or bipolar except shorter duration or too few symptoms)
- Unspecified depressive/bipolar disorder.

CHAPTER 5

ANXIETY, OBSESSIVE-COMPULSIVE, TRAUMA, AND STRESSOR-RELATED DISORDERS

Anxiety Disorders	50
Treatment guidelines	51
Pharmacotherapy	51
Psychotherapy	51
Panic Attacks	52
Panic Disorder	52
Agoraphobia	53
Specific Phobias	53
Social Anxiety Disorder (Social Phobia)	54
Selective Mutism	54
Separation Anxiety Disorder	55
Generalized Anxiety Disorder (GAD)	56
Obsessive-Compulsive and Related Disorders	57
Obsessive-Compulsive Disorder (OCD)	57
Body Dysmorphic Disorder	58
Hoarding Disorder	59
Trichotillomania (Hair-Pulling Disorder)	59
Excoriation (Skin-Picking) Disorder	60
Trauma and Stressor-Related Disorders	60
Posttraumatic Stress Disorder (PTSD) and Acute Stress Disorder	61
Adjustment Disorders	62

WARDS TIP

Assess for psychopathology if an individual's symptoms are causing **S**ocial and/or **O**ccupational **D**ysfunction (**SOD**).

Anxiety Disorders

Anxiety disorders are characterized by excessive or inappropriate fear or anxiety. *Fear* is manifested by a transient increase in sympathetic activity ("fight or flight" physiologic response, thoughts, feelings, behaviors) in a situation perceived to be dangerous or threatening. By contrast, *anxiety* involves apprehension regarding a future threat. The criteria for most anxiety disorders involve symptoms that cause **clinically significant distress** or **impairment in social and/or occupational functioning** (see Table 5-1).

- Anxiety disorders are caused by a combination of genetic, biological, environmental, and psychosocial factors.
- Primary anxiety disorders can only be diagnosed after determining that the signs and symptoms are **NOT due to the physiological effects of a substance, medication** (see Table 5-2), **or another medical condition** (see Table 5-3).
- Major neurotransmitter systems implicated: norepinephrine (NE), serotonin (5-HT), and gamma-aminobutyric acid (GABA).
- **Most common form of psychopathology.**
- More frequently seen in women compared to men, approximately 2:1 ratio.

TABLE 5-1. Signs and Symptoms of Anxiety

Constitutional	Fatigue, diaphoresis, shivering
Cardiac	Chest pain, palpitations, tachycardia, hypertension
Pulmonary	Shortness of breath, hyperventilation
Neurologic/musculoskeletal	Vertigo, light-headedness, paresthesias, tremors, insomnia, muscle tension
Gastrointestinal	Abdominal discomfort, anorexia, nausea, emesis, diarrhea, constipation

TABLE 5-2. Medications and Substances That Cause Anxiety

Alcohol	Intoxication/withdrawal
Sedatives, hypnotics, or anxiolytics	Withdrawal
Cannabis	Intoxication
Hallucinogens (PCP, LSD, MDMA)	Intoxication
Stimulants (amphetamines, cocaine)	Intoxication/withdrawal
Caffeine	Intoxication
Tobacco	Intoxication/withdrawal
Opioids	Withdrawal

Abbreviations: LSD, lysergic acid diethylamide; MDMA, 3,4-methylenedioxy methamphetamine; PCP, phencyclidine.

TABLE 5-3. Medical Conditions That Cause Anxiety

Neurologic	Epilepsy, migraines, brain tumors, multiple sclerosis, Huntington disease
Endocrine	Hyperthyroidism, hypoglycemia, pheochromocytoma, carcinoid syndrome
Metabolic	Vitamin B_{12} deficiency, electrolyte abnormalities, porphyria
Respiratory	Asthma, chronic obstructive pulmonary disease (COPD), hypoxia, pulmonary embolism (PE), pneumonia, pneumothorax
Cardiovascular	Congestive heart failure (CHF), angina, arrhythmia, myocardial infarction (MI)

Treatment guidelines

- Determine treatment course based on the severity of symptoms.
- Initiate **psychotherapy for mild anxiety**.
- Consider a **combination** of therapy and medication **for moderate to severe anxiety**.

Pharmacotherapy

- **Selective serotonin reuptake inhibitors (SSRIs)** (e.g., sertraline) and **serotonin-norepinephrine reuptake inhibitors (SNRIs)** (e.g., venlafaxine) are **first-line** medications.
- **Benzodiazepines** work quickly and effectively, but regular use results in dependence. Minimize the use, duration, and dose. Benzodiazepines should be avoided in patients with a history of substance use disorders, particularly alcohol. Mechanism of action: enhance activity of GABA at GABA-A receptor.
- In patients with comorbid substance use, consider non-addictive anxiolytic alternatives for PRN use, such as diphenhydramine, hydroxyzine, and gabapentin.
- **Buspirone** is a non-benzodiazepine anxiolytic which has partial agonist activity at the $5\text{-}HT_{1A}$ receptor. Due to minimal efficacy as monotherapy, buspirone is typically prescribed only as augmentation.
- **Beta-blockers (e.g., propranolol)** may be used to help control autonomic symptoms (e.g., palpitations, tachycardia, sweating) of **panic attacks** or **performance anxiety**.
- **Tricyclic antidepressants** (TCAs) and **monoamine oxidase inhibitors** (MAOIs) may be considered if first-line agents are not effective. Their side-effect profile makes them less tolerable and more dangerous.

Psychotherapy

- Many modalities of psychotherapy are helpful for patients suffering from anxiety disorders.
  - **Cognitive behavioral therapy (CBT)** has proven effective for anxiety disorders. CBT examines the relationship between anxiety-driven cognitions (thoughts), emotions, and behavior.
  - **Psychodynamic psychotherapy** facilitates insight into the development of anxiety symptoms, leading to more adaptive coping styles and subsequent improvement over time.

WARDS TIP

Late-onset anxiety symptoms without a prior history or family psychiatric history should increase suspicion of anxiety caused by another medical condition or substance use.

KEY FACT

If a patient has a comorbid depressive disorder, consider alternatives to benzodiazepines, as they may worsen depression.

WARDS TIP

Use *benzodiazepines* to temporarily *bridge* patients until long-term medication becomes effective.

WARDS TIP

SSRIs typically take about 4–6 weeks to become fully effective, and higher doses (than used in treating depression) are generally required.

WARDS TIP

Pharmacologic goal: Achieve symptomatic relief and continue treatment for at least 6 months before attempting to titrate off medications.

WARDS TIP

Medications can reduce symptoms enough so that a patient can participate in therapy. Therapy can help prevent relapse if medications are no longer prescribed.

KEY FACT

Symptoms of panic attacks
Da PANICS
Dizziness, **d**isconnectedness, **d**erealization (unreality), **d**epersonalization (detached from self)
Palpitations, **p**aresthesias
Abdominal distress
Numbness, **n**ausea
Intense fear of dying, losing control or "going crazy"
Chills, **c**hest pain
Sweating, **s**haking, **s**hortness of breath

WARDS TIP

Use the *B*s to *B*lock the *P*s: *B*eta-*B*lockers for *P*anic attacks and *P*erformance anxiety.

WARDS TIP

Smoking is a risk factor for panic attacks.

KEY FACT

When a patient presents with a panic attack, rule out potentially life-threatening medical conditions such as a heart attack, thyrotoxicosis, and thromboembolism.

WARDS TIP

A classic panic disorder case involves a woman who repeatedly visits the ER afraid she is dying when she experiences episodes of palpitations, diaphoresis, and shortness of breath. The patient has no prior medical history and the medical workup is negative.

WARDS TIP

Carefully screen patients with panic attacks for suicidality. They are at an increased risk for suicide attempts.

PANIC ATTACKS

A panic attack is a fear response involving a sudden onset of intense anxiety which may be triggered or occur spontaneously. Panic attacks peak within minutes and usually resolve within half an hour. Patients may continue to feel anxious for hours afterwards and believe they are experiencing a prolonged panic attack. Although classically associated with panic disorder, panic attacks can also be experienced with other psychiatric disorders and medical conditions.

PANIC DISORDER

Panic disorder is characterized by *spontaneous*, recurrent panic attacks. These attacks occur suddenly, *out of the blue*. Patients may also experience some panic attacks with a clear trigger. The frequency of attacks ranges from multiple times per day to a few monthly. Patients develop debilitating anticipatory anxiety about having future attacks—"fear of the fear."

Diagnosis and DSM-5 Criteria

- **Recurrent, *unexpected* panic attacks** without an identifiable trigger.
- One or more of panic attacks followed by ≥1 month of continuous worry about experiencing subsequent attacks or their consequences, and/or a maladaptive change in behaviors (e.g., avoidance of possible triggers).
- Not caused by the direct effects of a substance, another mental disorder, or another medical condition.

Etiology

- Genetic factors: Greater risk of panic disorder if a first-degree relative is affected.
- Psychosocial factors: ↑ incidence of stressors (especially loss) prior to onset of disorder; history of childhood physical or sexual abuse.

Epidemiology

- Lifetime prevalence: 4%.
- Higher rates in woman compared to men, approximately 2:1.
- Median age of onset: 20–24 years old.

Course and Prognosis

- Panic disorder has a chronic course with waxing and waning symptoms.
- Relapses are common with discontinuation of medication.
- Only a minority of patients have full remission of symptoms.
- Up to 65% of patients with panic disorder also have major depression.
- Other comorbid syndromes include other anxiety disorders (e.g., agoraphobia), bipolar disorder, and alcohol use disorder.

Treatment

Combination of CBT and Pharmacotherapy = most effective

- First-line: **SSRIs** (e.g., sertraline, citalopram, escitalopram).
- **SNRIs** (e.g., venlafaxine) are also efficacious.

- If above options are not effective, can try TCAs (e.g., clomipramine, imipramine).
- Can use benzodiazepines (e.g., clonazepam, lorazepam) as scheduled or PRN, especially until the other medications reach full efficacy.

AGORAPHOBIA

Agoraphobia is an intense fear of being in public places where escape or obtaining help may be difficult. It often develops with panic disorder. The course of the disorder is usually chronic. Avoidance behaviors may become as extreme as complete confinement to the home.

Diagnosis and DSM-5 Criteria

- Intense fear/anxiety about more than two situations due to concerns of difficulty escaping or obtaining help in case of panic or other humiliating symptoms:
  - Outside of the home alone.
  - Open spaces (e.g., bridges).
  - Enclosed places (e.g., stores).
  - Public transportation (e.g., trains).
  - Crowds/lines.
- The triggering situations cause fear/anxiety out of proportion to the potential danger posed, leading to endurance of intense anxiety, avoidance, or requiring a companion. This holds true even if the patient suffers from another medical condition such as inflammatory bowel disease (IBS) which may lead to embarrassing public scenarios.
- Symptoms cause significant social or occupational dysfunction.
- Symptoms last ≥6 months.
- Symptoms not better explained by another mental disorder.

Etiology

- Strong genetic factor: Heritability about 60%.
- Psychosocial factor: Onset frequently follows a traumatic event.

Course/Prognosis

- More than 50% of patients experience a panic attack prior to developing agoraphobia.
- Onset is usually before age 35.
- Course is persistent and chronic, with rare full remission.
- Comorbid diagnoses include other anxiety disorders, depressive disorders, and substance use disorders.

Treatment

- Similar approach as panic disorder: CBT and SSRIs (for panic symptoms).

SPECIFIC PHOBIAS

A phobia is defined as an **irrational fear that leads to endurance of the anxiety and/or avoidance** of the feared object or situation. A *specific phobia* is **an intense fear of a specific object or situation** (i.e., the phobic stimulus).

WARDS TIP

Start SSRIs or SNRIs at low doses and ↑ slowly because side effects may initially worsen anxiety, especially in panic disorder.

KEY FACT

Characteristic situations avoided in agoraphobia include bridges, crowds, buses, trains, or any open areas outside the home.

KEY FACT

Common Domains of Social Anxiety Disorder (Social Phobia):
- Speaking in public.
- Eating in public.
- Using public restrooms.

KEY FACT

Common Specific Phobias:
Animal—spiders, insects, dogs, snakes, and mice.
Natural environment—heights, storms, and water.
Situational—elevators, airplanes, enclosed spaces, and buses.
Blood-injection-injury—needles, injections, blood, invasive medical procedures, and injuries.

WARDS TIP

Patients with blood-injury-injection-specific phobia (fear of needles, etc.) may experience bradycardia and hypotension leading to vasovagal fainting.

KEY FACT

Substance use and depressive disorders frequently co-occur with phobias.

KEY FACT

Common Domains of Social Anxiety Disorder (Social Phobia):
- Speaking in public.
- Eating in public.
- Using public restrooms.

KEY FACT

Performance anxiety is often successfully treated with beta-blockers.

Diagnosis and DSM-5 Criteria

- Persistent, excessive fear elicited by a specific situation or object which is out of proportion to any actual danger/threat.
- Exposure to the situation triggers an immediate fear response.
- Situation or object is avoided when possible or tolerated with intense anxiety.
- Symptoms cause significant social or occupational dysfunction.
- Duration ≥6 months.
- Symptoms not solely due to another mental disorder, substance (medication or drug), or another medical condition.

Epidemiology

- Phobias are the **most common psychiatric disorder** in women and **second most common in men** (substance-related is first).
- Lifetime prevalence of specific phobia: >10%.
- Mean age of onset for specific phobia is 10 years.
- Specific phobia rates are higher in women compared to men (2:1) but vary depending on the type of stimulus.

Treatment

- Treatment of choice: CBT.

SOCIAL ANXIETY DISORDER (SOCIAL PHOBIA)

Social anxiety disorder (social phobia) is the **fear of scrutiny by others or fear of acting in a humiliating or embarrassing way**. The phobia may develop in the wake of negative or traumatic encounters with the stimulus. Social situations causing significant anxiety may be avoided altogether, resulting in social and academic/occupational impairment.

The diagnostic criteria for **social anxiety disorder (social phobia)** are similar to specific phobia except the phobic stimulus is related to social scrutiny and negative evaluation. The patients fear embarrassment, humiliation, and rejection. This fear may be limited to performance or public speaking, which may be routinely encountered in the patient's occupation or academic pursuit.

Epidemiology

- Median age of onset for social anxiety disorder is 13 years.
- Social anxiety disorder occurs equally in men and women.

Treatment

- Treatment of choice: CBT.
- First-line medication, if needed: SSRIs (e.g., sertraline, fluoxetine) or SNRIs (e.g., venlafaxine) for debilitating symptoms.
- Benzodiazepines (e.g., clonazepam, lorazepam) can be used as scheduled or PRN.
- **Beta-blockers** (e.g., atenolol, **propranolol**) for performance anxiety/public speaking.

SELECTIVE MUTISM

Selective mutism is a rare condition characterized by a failure to speak in specific situations for at least 1 month, despite the intact ability to comprehend and use language. Symptom onset typically starts during childhood. The majority of these patients suffer from anxiety, particularly social anxiety as the mutism manifests in social settings. The patients may remain completely silent or whisper. They may use nonverbal means of communication, such as writing or gesturing.

Diagnosis and DSM-5 Criteria

- Consistent failure to speak in select social situations (e.g., school) despite speech ability in other scenarios.
- Mutism is not due to a language difficulty or a communication disorder.
- Symptoms cause significant impairment in academic, occupational, or social functioning.
- Symptoms last >1 month (extending beyond first month of school).

Treatment

- Psychotherapy: CBT, family therapy.
- Medications: SSRIs (especially with comorbid social anxiety disorder).

SEPARATION ANXIETY DISORDER

As part of normal human development, infants become distressed when they are separated from their primary caregiver. *Stranger anxiety* begins around 6 months and peaks around 9 months, while *separation anxiety* typically emerges by 1 year of age and peaks by 18 months. When the anxiety due to separation becomes extreme or developmentally inappropriate, it is considered pathologic. Separation anxiety disorder may be preceded by a stressful life event.

WARDS TIP

Separation anxiety may lead to complaints of somatic symptoms to avoid school/work.

Diagnosis and DSM-5 Criteria

Excessive and developmentally inappropriate fear/anxiety regarding **separation from attachment figures**, with at least three of the following:

- Separation from attachment figures leads to extreme distress.
- Excessive worry about loss of or harm to attachment figures.
- Excessive worry about experiencing an event that leads to separation from attachment figures.
- Reluctance to leave home, or attend school or work.
- Reluctance to be alone.
- Reluctance to sleep alone or away from home.
- Complaints of physical symptoms when separated from major attachment figures.
- Nightmares of separation and refusal to sleep without proximity to attachment figure.
- Lasts for ≥4 weeks in children/adolescents and ≥6 months in adults.
- Symptoms cause significant social, academic, or occupational dysfunction.
- Symptoms not due to another mental disorder.

Treatment

- Psychotherapy: CBT, family therapy.
- Medications: SSRIs can be effective as an adjunct to therapy.

A 24-year-old law student presents to an outpatient psychiatry clinic accompanied by her husband because she feels overwhelmed with worry "about everything." She is stressed about her academic workload and upcoming exams. She has had trouble falling asleep and feels chronically fatigued. The patient complains of frequent headaches and has difficulty concentrating on her assignments.

The patient's husband describes her as "a worrier. She'll worry about me getting into an accident, losing my job, not making enough money—the list goes on and on."

The patient reports that she has always had some degree of anxiety, but previously found it motivating. Over the last year since starting law school, her symptoms have become debilitating.

What is the most likely diagnosis?

With the patient's history of *excessive worrying* about *everything*, the most likely diagnosis is generalized anxiety disorder (GAD). Like many patients with GAD, she is described as a *worrier*. She reports typical associated symptoms: insomnia, fatigue, and impaired concentration. Her symptoms have been present for over *6 months*.

What is the next step?

A complete physical exam and medical workup should be performed to rule out other medical conditions or substance use contributing to or causing her anxiety symptoms.

What are treatment options?

Treatment options for GAD include psychotherapy (usually CBT) and pharmacotherapy (typically SSRIs). A combination of both modalities may achieve better remission rates than either treatment alone.

WARDS TIP

GAD Mnemonic
Worry WARTS
Wound up, **w**orn-out
Absent-minded
Restless
Tense
Sleepless

WARDS TIP

For patients with anxiety, evaluate for caffeine use and recommend significant reduction or elimination.

WARDS TIP

Exercise can significantly reduce anxiety.

WARDS TIP

The worries associated with *generalized* anxiety disorder are free-floating across various areas, as opposed to being fixed on a specific trigger.

GENERALIZED ANXIETY DISORDER (GAD)

Patients with GAD have persistent, excessive anxiety about many aspects of their daily lives. Often they experience somatic symptoms including fatigue and muscle tension. Not uncommonly, these physical complaints lead patients to initially present to a primary care physician.

Diagnosis and DSM-5 Criteria

- Excessive, anxiety/worry about various daily events/activities ≥6 months.
- Difficulty controlling the worry.
- Associated ≥3 symptoms: restlessness, fatigue, impaired concentration, irritability, muscle tension, insomnia.
- Symptoms are not caused by the direct effects of a substance, or another mental disorder or medical condition.
- Symptoms cause significant social or occupational dysfunction.

Epidemiology/Etiology

- Lifetime prevalence: 5–9%.
- GAD rates higher in women compared to men (2:1).
- One-third of risk for developing GAD is genetic.

Course/Prognosis

- Symptoms of worry begin in childhood.
- Median age of onset of GAD: 30 years.
- Course is chronic, with waxing and waning symptoms.

- Rates of full remission are low.
- GAD is highly comorbid with other anxiety and depressive disorders.

Treatment

The most effective treatment approach combines psychotherapy and pharmacotherapy:

- CBT.
- SSRIs (e.g., sertraline, citalopram) or SNRIs (e.g., venlafaxine).
- Can also consider a short-term course of benzodiazepines or augmentation with buspirone.
- Much less commonly used medications are TCAs and MAOIs.

Obsessive-Compulsive and Related Disorders

OBSESSIVE-COMPULSIVE DISORDER (OCD)

Obsessive-compulsive disorder (OCD) is characterized by obsessions and/or compulsions that are time-consuming, distressing, and impairing. **Obsessions** are recurrent, intrusive, undesired thoughts that increase anxiety. Patients may attempt to relieve this anxiety by performing **compulsions**, which are repetitive behaviors or mental rituals. Anxiety may increase when a patient resists acting out a compulsion.

Patients with OCD have varying degrees of insight.

Diagnosis and DSM-5 Criteria

- Experiencing obsessions and/or compulsions that are time-consuming (e.g., >1 hr/day) or cause significant distress or dysfunction.
  - **Obsessions:** Recurrent, intrusive, anxiety-provoking thoughts, images, or urges that the patient attempts to suppress, ignore, or neutralize by some other thought or action (i.e., by performing a compulsion).
  - **Compulsions:** Repetitive behaviors or mental acts the patient feels driven to perform in response to an obsession, or a rule aimed at stress reduction or disaster prevention. The behaviors are excessive and/or not realistically connected to what they are meant to prevent.
- Not caused by the direct effects of a substance, another mental illness, or another medical condition.

Epidemiology

- Lifetime prevalence: 2–3%.
- No gender difference in prevalence overall.

Etiology

- Significant genetic component: Higher rates of OCD in first-degree relatives and monozygotic twins than in the general population. Higher rate of OCD in first-degree relatives with Tourette's disorder.

Course/Prognosis

- Chronic, with waxing and waning symptoms.
- Less than 20% remission rate without treatment.
- Suicidal ideation in 50%, attempts in 25% of patients with OCD.
- High comorbidity with other anxiety disorders, depressive or bipolar disorder, obsessive-compulsive personality disorder, and tic disorder.

KEY FACT

Compulsions can often take the form of repeated checking or counting.

KEY FACT

Patients with OCD often initially seek help from primary care and other nonpsychiatric providers for help with the consequences of compulsions (e.g., excessive washing).

KEY FACT

The triad of "uncontrollable urges"— OCD, ADHD, and tic disorder—are usually first seen in children or adolescents.

KEY FACT

Common Patterns of Obsessions and Compulsions

Obsessions	Compulsions
Contamination	Cleaning or avoidance of contaminant
Doubt or harm	Checking multiple times to avoid potential danger
Symmetry	Ordering or counting
Intrusive, taboo thoughts	With or without related compulsion

KEY FACT

Differentiating OCD and obsessive-compulsive personality disorder (OCPD):
- Individuals with OCPD are obsessed with details, control, and perfectionism; they are not intruded upon by unwanted preoccupations nor compelled to carry out compulsions.
- OCD patients are *dis*tressed by their symptoms (ego-*dys*tonic).

Treatment

Utilize a combination of psychopharmacology and CBT

CBT focuses on *exposure and response prevention*: prolonged, graded exposure to ritual-eliciting stimulus and prevention of the relieving compulsion.

- First-line medication: SSRIs (e.g., sertraline, fluoxetine), typically at higher doses.
- Second-line agents: SNRIs (e.g., venlafaxine) or the most serotonin selective **TCA, clomipramine.**
- Can augment with atypical antipsychotics.
- Last resort: In debilitating, treatment-resistant cases, can use psychosurgery (cingulotomy) or electroconvulsive therapy (ECT).

BODY DYSMORPHIC DISORDER

- Patients with body dysmorphic disorder are preoccupied with nonexistent or minor physical defects that they regard as severe, grotesque, and repulsive.
- These individuals spend significant time trying to correct perceived flaws with makeup, dermatological procedures, or plastic surgery.

Diagnosis and DSM-5 Criteria

- Preoccupation with one or more perceived defects or flaws in physical appearance that are not observable by or appear slight to others.
- In response to the appearance concerns, repetitive behaviors (e.g., skin picking, excessive grooming) or mental acts (e.g., comparing appearance to others) are performed.
- Preoccupation causes significant distress or impairment in functioning.
- Appearance preoccupation is not better accounted for by concerns with body fat/weight in an eating disorder.

Epidemiology

- May be slightly more common in women than men.
- Prevalence elevated in those with high rates of childhood abuse and neglect
- Increased risk in first-degree relatives of patients with OCD.
- Higher prevalence in dermatologic and cosmetic surgery patients.
- Mean age of onset: 15 years.

Course/Prognosis

- The onset is usually gradual, beginning in early adolescence. Symptoms tend to be chronic.
- Surgical or dermatological procedures are routinely unsuccessful in satisfying the patient.
- High rate of suicidal ideation and attempts.
- Comorbidity with major depression, social anxiety disorder (social phobia), and OCD.

Treatment

- SSRIs and/or CBT may reduce the obsessive and compulsive symptoms in many patients.

HOARDING DISORDER

Diagnosis and DSM-5 Criteria
- Persistent difficulty discarding possessions, regardless of value.
- Difficulty is due to need to save the items and distress associated with discarding them.
- Results in accumulation of possessions that congest/clutter living areas and compromise use.
- Hoarding causes clinically significant distress or impairment in social, occupational, or other areas of functioning.
- Hoarding is not attributable to another medical condition or another mental disorder.

Epidemiology/Etiology
- Point prevalence of significant hoarding is 2–6%.
- Hoarding is three times more prevalent in older population.
- Onset often preceded by stressful and traumatic events.
- Fifty percent of individuals with hoarding have a relative who also hoards.

Course/Prognosis
- Hoarding behavior begins in early teens.
- Hoarding tends to worsen.
- Usually chronic course.
- Seventy-five percent of individuals have comorbid mood (MDD) or anxiety disorder (social anxiety disorder).
- Twenty percent of individuals have comorbid OCD.

Treatment
- Very difficult to treat.
- Specialized CBT for hoarding.
- SSRIs can be used.

TRICHOTILLOMANIA (HAIR-PULLING DISORDER)

Diagnosis and DSM-5 Criteria
- Recurrent pulling out of one's hair, resulting in hair loss.
- Repeated attempts to decrease or stop hair pulling.
- Causes significant distress or impairment in daily functioning.
- Hair pulling or hair loss is not due to another medical condition or psychiatric disorder.
- Usually involves the scalp, eyebrows, or eyelashes. May include facial, axillary, and pubic hair.

Epidemiology/Etiology
- Lifetime prevalence: 1–2% of the adult population.
- More common in women than in men (10:1 ratio).
- Onset usually at puberty. Frequently associated with a stressful event.
- Etiology may involve biological, genetic, and environmental factors.
- Increased incidence of comorbid OCD, major depressive disorder, and excoriation (skin-picking) disorder.

- Course may be chronic with waxing and waning periods. Adult onset is generally more difficult to treat.

Treatment

- Treatment includes SSRIs, second-generation antipsychotics, lithium, or *N*-acetylcysteine.
- Specialized types of cognitive-behavior therapy (e.g., habit reversal training).

EXCORIATION (SKIN-PICKING) DISORDER

Diagnosis and DSM-5 Criteria

- Recurrent skin picking resulting in lesions.
- Repeated attempts to decrease or stop skin picking.
- Causes significant distress or impairment in daily functioning.
- Skin picking is not due to a substance, another medical condition, or another psychiatric disorder.

Epidemiology/Etiology

- Lifetime prevalence: 1.4% of the adult population.
- More than 75% of cases are women.
- More common in individuals with OCD and first-degree family members.

Course/Prognosis

- Skin picking begins in adolescence.
- Course is chronic with waxing and waning periods if untreated.
- Comorbidity with OCD, trichotillomania, and MDD.

Treatment

- Specialized types of cognitive-behavior therapy (e.g., habit reversal training).
- SSRIs have shown some benefit.

Trauma and Stressor-Related Disorders

A 19-year-old freshman is brought to the ER by her college dorm mate. The dorm mate reports that the patient has been isolating herself, crying in their room, and screaming in her sleep. The dorm mate states, "this isn't like her at all" and discloses concern that something happened at a recent party they attended 5 weeks ago. "She hasn't been the same since." The patient is reluctant to talk at first. Eventually she discloses that she was forced to have sex with one of the fraternity brothers. Since that night, she has experienced intrusive thoughts and nightmares. The patient fears she will be victimized again and feels on edge. She has avoided most places where she might encounter the rapist. She has hardly left her dorm room, even to attend class. Her sense of shame and embarrassment has kept her emotionally isolated.

What is the most likely diagnosis?

The patient has been suffering from symptoms of PTSD for the last 5 weeks after being raped: low mood, avoidance, hypervigilance, intrusive thoughts, and nightmares.

TABLE 5-4. Posttraumatic Stress Disorder and Acute Stress Disorder

Posttraumatic Stress Disorder	Acute Stress Disorder
Trauma occurred at any time in past	Trauma occurred <1 month ago
Symptoms last >1 month	Symptoms last <1 month

POSTTRAUMATIC STRESS DISORDER (PTSD) AND ACUTE STRESS DISORDER

Posttraumatic stress disorder (PTSD) is characterized by the development of multiple symptoms after exposure to one or more traumatic events: intrusive symptoms (e.g., nightmares, flashbacks), avoidance, negative alterations in thoughts and mood, and increased arousal. The symptoms last for at least a month and may occur immediately after the trauma or with delayed expression.

Acute stress disorder is diagnosed in patients who experience a major traumatic event and suffer from similar symptoms as PTSD (see Table 5-4) but for a shorter duration. The onset of symptoms occurs within 1 month of the trauma and symptoms last for less than 1 month.

Diagnosis and DSM-5 Criteria

- Exposure to actual or threatened death, serious injury, or sexual violence by directly experiencing or witnessing the trauma.
- Recurrent intrusions of re-experiencing the event via memories, nightmares, or dissociative reactions (e.g., flashbacks); intense distress at exposure to cues relating to the trauma; or physiological reactions to cues relating to the trauma.
- Active avoidance of triggering stimuli (e.g., memories, feelings, people, places, objects) associated with the trauma.
- At least two of the following negative cognitions/mood: dissociative amnesia, negative feelings of self/others/world, self-blame, negative emotions (e.g., fear, horror, anger, guilt), anhedonia, feelings of detachment/estrangement, inability to experience positive emotions.
- At least two of the following symptoms of increased arousal/reactivity: hypervigilance, exaggerated startle response, irritability/angry outbursts, impaired concentration, insomnia.
- Symptoms not caused by the direct effects of a substance or another medical condition.
- Symptoms result in significant impairment in social or occupational functioning.
- The presentation differs in children <7 years of age.

Epidemiology/Etiology

- Lifetime prevalence of PTSD: >8%.
- Higher prevalence in women, most likely due to greater risk of exposure to traumatic events, particularly rape and other forms of interpersonal violence.
- Exposure to prior trauma, especially during childhood, is a risk factor for developing PTSD.

Course/Prognosis

- PTSD usually begins within 3 months after the trauma.
- Symptoms may manifest after a delayed expression.
- Fifty percent of patients with PTSD have complete recovery within 3 months.

KEY FACT

Use **P**razo**SiN**
in **P**TSD to **S**top **N**ightmares

WARDS TIP

Etiology of PTSD: TRAUMA
Traumatic event
Reexperience
Avoidance
Unable to function
Month or more of symptoms
Arousal increased

WARDS TIP

Cognitive processing therapy is a modified form of cognitive-behavioral therapy in which thoughts, feelings, and meanings of the event are revisited and questioned.

WARDS TIP

Addictive medications such as benzodiazepines should be avoided in the treatment of PTSD because of the high rate of comorbid substance use disorders.

KEY FACT

Posttraumatic stress disorder (PTSD) stressor = life threatening!
Adjustment disorder stressor ≠ life threatening.

- Symptoms tend to diminish with older age.
- Eighty percent of patients with PTSD have a comorbid mental disorder (e.g., MDD, bipolar disorder, anxiety disorder, substance use disorder).

Treatment
- **Pharmacological**
  - First-line antidepressants: SSRIs (e.g., sertraline, citalopram) or SNRIs (e.g., venlafaxine).
  - Prazosin, α_1-receptor antagonist, targets **nightmares** and hypervigilance.
  - May augment with atypical (second-generation) antipsychotics in severe cases.
- **Psychotherapy**
  - Specialized forms of CBT (e.g., exposure therapy, cognitive processing therapy).
  - Supportive and psychodynamic therapy.
  - Couples/family therapy.

ADJUSTMENT DISORDERS

Adjustment disorders occur when behavioral or emotional symptoms develop after a non-life-threatening, stressful life event (e.g., divorce, death of a loved one, or loss of a job).

Diagnosis and DSM-5 Criteria
1. Development of emotional or behavioral symptoms within 3 months in response to an identifiable stressful life event. These symptoms produce either:
   - Excessive distress in relation to the event.
   - Significant impairment in daily functioning.
2. The symptoms are not those of normal bereavement.
3. Symptoms resolve within 6 months after stressor has terminated.
4. The stress-related disturbance does not meet criteria for another mental disorder.

Subtypes: Based on a predominance of either depressed mood, anxiety, mixed anxiety and depression, disturbance of conduct (such as aggression), or mixed disturbance of emotions and conduct.

Epidemiology
- Five percent to twenty percent of patients in outpatient mental health clinics have an adjustment disorder.
- May occur at any age.

Etiology
- Triggered by psychosocial factors.

Prognosis
May be chronic if the stressor is chronic or recurrent.

Treatment
- Supportive psychotherapy.
- Group therapy.
- If necessary, pharmacotherapy can target associated symptoms (insomnia, anxiety, or depression).

CHAPTER 6

PERSONALITY DISORDERS

Definition	64
Diagnosis and DSM-5 Criteria	64
Clusters	64
Etiology	64
Treatment	65
Cluster A	65
Paranoid Personality Disorder (PPD)	65
Schizoid Personality Disorder	66
Schizotypal Personality Disorder	67
Cluster B	68
Antisocial Personality Disorder	69
Borderline Personality Disorder (BPD)	70
Histrionic Personality Disorder (HPD)	71
Narcissistic Personality Disorder (NPD)	72
Cluster C	73
Avoidant Personality Disorder	73
Dependent Personality Disorder (DPD)	74
Obsessive-Compulsive Personality Disorder (OCPD)	75
Personality Change Due to Another Medical Condition	76
Other Specified Personality Disorder	76
Unspecified Personality Disorder	76

WARDS TIP

Many people have odd tendencies and quirks. These are not pathological unless they cause significant distress or impairment in daily functioning.

KEY FACT

Ego-syntonic refers to feelings, thoughts, and/or behaviors that are acceptable to the self; that are consistent with one's fundamental personality. *Ego-dystonic* refers to feelings, thoughts, and/or behaviors that are distressing, unacceptable, or inconsistent with one's self-concept.

WARDS TIP

Personality disorder criteria—
CAPRI
Cognition
Affect
Personal **R**elations
Impulse control

Definition

Personality is one's set of stable, predictable, emotional, and behavioral traits. Personality *disorders* involve enduring patterns of inner experience and behavior that deviate markedly from expectations of an individual's culture. They are pervasive, **maladaptive,** and cause significant impairment in social or occupational functioning. Patients with personality disorders often lack insight about their problems; their symptoms are either **ego-syntonic** or viewed as immutable. In addition, individuals with personality disorders have significant comorbidity with other mental disorders.

DIAGNOSIS AND DSM-5 CRITERIA

1. Enduring pattern of behavior/inner experience that deviates from the person's culture and is manifested in two or more of the following ways:
   - Cognition
   - Affect
   - Interpersonal functioning
   - Impulse control
2. The pattern:
   - Is **pervasive** and **inflexible** in a broad range of situations.
   - Is **stable** and has an onset no later than adolescence or early adulthood.
   - Leads to significant distress in functioning.
   - Is not accounted for by another mental/medical illness or by use of a substance.

The international prevalence of personality disorders is 6–11%. Personality disorders vary by gender. Many patients with personality disorders will meet the criteria for more than one disorder; they should be classified as having all of the disorders for which they qualify.

Clusters

Personality disorders are divided into the following three clusters:

- **Cluster A**—schizoid, schizotypal, and paranoid:
  - Patients seem eccentric, peculiar, or withdrawn.
  - Familial association with psychotic disorders.
- **Cluster B**—antisocial, borderline, histrionic, and narcissistic:
  - Patients seem emotional, dramatic, or inconsistent.
  - Familial association with mood disorders.
- **Cluster C**—avoidant, dependent, and obsessive-compulsive:
  - Patients seem anxious or fearful.
  - Familial association with anxiety disorders.

Other specified/unspecified personality disorder includes characteristics of a personality disorder that do not meet full criteria for any of the other personality disorders.

ETIOLOGY

- Biological, genetic, and psychosocial factors during childhood and adolescence contribute to the development of personality disorders.
- The prevalence of some personality disorders in monozygotic twins is several times higher than in dizygotic twins.

TREATMENT

- Personality disorders are generally very difficult to treat, especially since few patients are aware that they need help. The disorders tend to be chronic and lifelong.
- In general, pharmacologic treatment has limited usefulness (see individual exceptions below) except in treating comorbid mental conditions (e.g., major depressive disorder).
- Psychotherapy is usually the most helpful.

Cluster A

These patients are perceived as eccentric or odd by others and can have psychotic symptoms (see Table 6-1).

PARANOID PERSONALITY DISORDER (PPD)

Patients with paranoid personality disorder (PPD) have a pervasive distrust and suspiciousness of others and often interpret motives as malevolent. They tend to blame their own problems on others and seem angry and hostile. They are often characterized as being pathologically jealous, which leads them to think that their sexual partners or spouses are cheating on them.

Diagnosis and DSM-5 Criteria

- Diagnosis requires a general distrust of others, beginning by early adulthood and present in a variety of contexts.

TABLE 6-1. Cluster A Personality Disorders and Classic Clinical Examples

Personality Disorder	Clinical Example
Paranoid personality disorder	A 30-year-old man says his wife has been cheating on him because he does not have a good enough job to provide for her needs. He also claims that on his previous job, his boss laid him off because he did a better job than his boss. He has initiated several lawsuits. Refuses couples therapy because he believes the therapist will side with his wife. Believes neighbors are critical of him.
Schizoid personality disorder	A 45-year-old scientist works in the lab most of the day and has no friends, according to his coworkers. Has not been able to keep his job because of failure to collaborate with others. He expresses no desire to make friends and is content with his single life. He has no evidence of a thought disorder.
Schizotypal personality disorder	A 35-year-old man dresses in a wizard costume every weekend with friends as part of a live action role-playing community. He spends a great deal of time on his computers set up in his basement for video games and to "detect the presence of extraterrestrial communications in space." He has no auditory or visual hallucinations. He is lonely and sad, desiring an intimate relationship.

- At least four of the following must also be present:
  1. Suspicion (without evidence) that others are exploiting or deceiving him or her.
  2. Preoccupation with doubts of loyalty or trustworthiness of friends or acquaintances.
  3. Reluctance to confide in others.
  4. Interpretation of benign remarks as threatening or demeaning.
  5. Persistence of grudges.
  6. Perception of attacks on his or her character that is not apparent to others; quick to counterattack.
  7. Suspicions regarding fidelity of spouse or partner.

Epidemiology
- Prevalence: 2–4%.
- More commonly diagnosed in men than in women.
- Higher incidence in family members of schizophrenics.
- This personality disorder may be misdiagnosed in minority groups, immigrants, and deaf individuals.

Differential Diagnosis
- *Schizophrenia:* Unlike patients with schizophrenia, patients with PPD *do not have any fixed delusions and are not frankly psychotic,* although they may have transient psychosis under stressful situations.
- *Social disenfranchisement and social isolation:* Without a social support system, persons can react with suspicion to others. The differential in favor of the PPD can be assisted by the assessment of others in close contact with the person, who may identify what they consider as excess suspicion.

Course and Prognosis
- The disorder usually has a chronic course, causing lifelong marital and job-related problems.

Treatment
- Psychotherapy is the treatment of choice, although, as stated above, patients rarely initiate treatment.
- Group psychotherapy should be avoided due to mistrust and misinterpretation of others' statements.
- Patients may also benefit from a short course of antipsychotics for transient psychosis.

SCHIZOID PERSONALITY DISORDER

Patients with schizoid personality disorder have a lifelong pattern of social withdrawal. They are often perceived as eccentric and reclusive. They are quiet, unsociable, and have a constricted affect. They have *no desire for close relationships* and prefer to be alone.

KEY FACT

Unlike with avoidant personality disorder, patients with schizoid personality disorder *prefer* to be alone.

Diagnosis and DSM-5 Criteria
- A pattern of voluntary social withdrawal and restricted range of emotional expression, beginning by early adulthood and present in a variety of contexts.
- Four or more of the following must also be present:
  1. Neither enjoying nor desiring close relationships (including family).
  2. Generally choosing solitary activities.
  3. Little (if any) interest in sexual activity with another person.
  4. Taking pleasure in few activities (if any).

5. Few close friends or confidants (if any).
6. Indifference to praise or criticism.
7. Emotional coldness, detachment, or flattened affect.

Epidemiology
- Prevalence: 3–5%.
- Diagnosed more often in men than women.
- May be increased prevalence of schizoid personality disorder in relatives of individuals with schizophrenia.

Differential Diagnosis
- *Schizophrenia:* Unlike patients with schizophrenia, patients with schizoid personality disorder do not have any fixed delusions or hallucinations.
- *Schizotypal personality disorder:* Patients with schizoid personality disorder do not have the same eccentric behavior or magical thinking seen in patients with schizotypal personality disorder. Schizotypal patients are more similar to schizophrenic patients in terms of odd perception, thought, and behavior.

Course
Usually chronic course.

Treatment
- Lack insight for individual psychotherapy, and may find group therapy threatening; may benefit from day programs or drop-in centers.
- Antidepressants if comorbid major depression is diagnosed.

SCHIZOTYPAL PERSONALITY DISORDER

Patients with schizotypal personality disorder have a pervasive pattern of eccentric behavior and peculiar thought patterns. They are often perceived as strange and odd. The disorder was developed out of the observation that certain family traits predominate in first-degree relatives of those with schizophrenia.

Diagnosis and DSM-5 Criteria
- A pattern of social deficits marked by eccentric behavior, cognitive or perceptual distortions, and discomfort with close relationships, beginning by early adulthood and present in a variety of contexts.
- Five or more of the following must be present:
  1. Ideas of reference (excluding delusions of reference).
  2. Odd beliefs or magical thinking, inconsistent with cultural norms.
  3. Unusual perceptual experiences (such as bodily illusions).
  4. Suspiciousness.
  5. Inappropriate or restricted affect.
  6. Odd or eccentric appearance or behavior.
  7. Few close friends or confidants.
  8. Odd thinking or speech (vague, stereotyped, etc.).
  9. Excessive social anxiety.
- Magical thinking may include:
  - Belief in clairvoyance or telepathy.
  - Bizarre fantasies or preoccupations.
  - Belief in superstitions.
- Odd behaviors may include involvement in cults or strange religious practices.

Epidemiology

Prevalence: 4%.

Differential Diagnosis

- *Schizophrenia:* Unlike patients with schizophrenia, patients with schizotypal personality disorder are not frankly psychotic (though they can become transiently so under stress), nor do they have fixed delusions.
- *Schizoid personality disorder:* Patients with schizoid personality disorder do not have the same eccentric behavior seen in patients with schizotypal personality disorder.

Course

- Course is chronic, with a small minority developing schizophrenia.
- Premorbid personality type for a patient with schizophrenia.

Treatment

- Psychotherapy is the treatment of choice to help develop social skills training.
- Short course of low-dose antipsychotics if necessary (for transient psychosis). Antipsychotics may help decrease social anxiety and suspicion in interpersonal relationships.

Cluster B

Includes antisocial, borderline, histrionic, and narcissistic personality disorders. These patients are often emotional, impulsive, and dramatic (Table 6-2).

TABLE 6-2. Cluster B Personality Disorders and Classic Clinical Examples

Personality Disorder	Clinical Example
Antisocial personality disorder	A 30-year-old unemployed man has been accused of killing three senior citizens after robbing them. He is surprisingly charming in the interview. In his adolescence, he was arrested several times for stealing cars and assaulting other kids.
Borderline personality disorder	A 23-year-old medical student attempted to cut her wrist because things did not work out with a man she had been dating over the past 3 weeks. She states that guys are jerks and "not worth her time." She often feels that she is "alone in this world."
Histrionic personality disorder	A 33-year-old scantily clad woman comes to your office complaining that her fever feels like "she is burning in hell." She vividly describes how the fever has affected her work as a teacher.
Narcissistic personality disorder	A 48-year-old company CEO is rushed to the ED after an automobile accident. He does not let the residents operate on him and requests the Chief of trauma surgery because he is "vital to the company." He makes several business phone calls in the ED to stay on "top of his game."

PERSONALITY DISORDERS CHAPTER 6

> Mr. Harris is a 35-year-old man with no prior psychiatric history who was arrested for assaulting his pregnant girlfriend. While in jail, he reports feeling depressed, and you are called in for a psychiatric evaluation. Mr. Harris is cooperative during the evaluation and presents as friendly and likeable. He reports that he is innocent of his charges and expresses feeling sad and tearful since his incarceration 2 days ago. He requests that you transfer him to the mental health unit at the correctional facility. However, you perform a thorough evaluation, and you do not find symptoms suggestive of a mood or psychotic disorder. When asked if he has been incarcerated before, he reports a history of multiple arrests and convictions for robbery and gun possession. He reports that he is unemployed because he has been "in and out of jail" during the past 5 years. He provides rationalizations for his limited involvement in these past crimes and does not appear remorseful.
>
> Mr. Harris reveals a pattern of repeated fights since childhood and says that he quit school while in the ninth grade after being suspended for smoking pot on school grounds. Mr. Harris reports that throughout his childhood he bullied others, and laughs when recounting an episode during which he threw his cat against the wall to see it bounce back. He denies any family history of psychiatric illnesses, but reports that his father is currently incarcerated for drug trafficking.
>
> *What is his diagnosis?*
>
> Mr. Harris's diagnosis is antisocial personality disorder. His history shows a pervasive pattern of disregard for and violation of the rights of others since age 15, and there is evidence of conduct disorder with onset before age 15 years. Remember that, although it is common, not all criminals have antisocial personality disorder.
>
> *What are some associated findings?*
>
> Antisocial personality disorder is more prevalent in males, is associated with low socioeconomic background, and has a genetic predisposition. It has been found that the children of parents with antisocial personality disorder have an increased risk for this disorder, somatic symptom disorder, and substance use disorders.

ANTISOCIAL PERSONALITY DISORDER

Patients diagnosed with antisocial personality disorder often exploit and violate the rights of others, and break rules to meet their own needs. They lack empathy, compassion, and remorse for their actions. They are impulsive, deceitful, and often violate the law. They are frequently skilled at reading social cues and can appear charming and normal to others who meet them for the first time and do not know their history.

Diagnosis and DSM-5 Criteria

- Pattern of disregard for and violation of the rights of others since age 15.
- Patients must be **at least 18 years old** for this diagnosis; history of behavior as a child/adolescent must be consistent with **conduct disorder** (see Chap. 10, "Psychiatric Disorders in Children").
- Three or more of the following should be present:
    1. Failure to conform to social norms by committing unlawful acts.
    2. Deceitfulness/repeated lying/manipulating others for personal gain.

WARDS TIP

Symptoms of antisocial personality disorder—
CORRUPT
Cannot follow law
Obligations ignored
Remorselessness
Reckless disregard for safety
Underhanded (deceitful)
Planning deficit (impulsive)
Temper (irritable, aggressive)

KEY FACT

Antisocial personality disorder begins in childhood as conduct disorder. Patient may have a history of being abused (physically or sexually) as a child or a history of hurting animals or starting fires. It is often associated with violations of the law.

WARDS TIP

The name borderline comes from the patient's being on the borderline of neurosis and psychosis.

WARDS TIP

Symptoms of borderline personality disorder—
IMPULSIVE
Impulsive
Moody
Paranoid under stress
Unstable self-image
Labile, intense relationships
Suicidal
Inappropriate anger
Vulnerable to abandonment
Emptiness

---

3. Impulsivity/failure to plan ahead.
4. Irritability and aggressiveness/repeated fights or assaults.
5. Recklessness and disregard for safety of self or others.
6. Irresponsibility/failure to sustain work or honor financial obligations.
7. Lack of remorse for actions.

Epidemiology

- Prevalence: 3% in men and 1% in women.
- Males with alcoholic parents are at increased risk.
- There is a higher incidence in poor urban areas and in prisoners but no racial difference.
- Genetic component: Increased risk among first-degree relatives.

Differential Diagnosis

Drug abuse: It is necessary to ascertain which came first. Patients who began abusing drugs before their antisocial behavior started may have behavior attributable to the effects of their addiction.

Course

- Usually has a chronic course, but some improvement of symptoms may occur as the patient ages.
- Many patients have multiple somatic complaints, and coexistence of substance use disorders and/or major depression is common.
- There is increased morbidity from substance use, trauma, suicide, or homicide.

Treatment

- Psychotherapy is generally ineffective.
- Pharmacotherapy may be used to treat symptoms of anxiety or depression, but use caution due to high addictive potential of these patients.

BORDERLINE PERSONALITY DISORDER (BPD)

Patients with borderline personality disorder (BPD) have unstable moods, behaviors, and interpersonal relationships. They fear abandonment and have poorly formed identity. Relationships begin with intense attachments and end with the slightest conflict. Aggression is common. They are impulsive and may have a history of repeated suicide attempts/gestures or episodes of self-mutilation. They have higher rates of childhood physical, emotional, and sexual abuse than the general population.

Diagnosis and DSM-5 Criteria

- Pervasive pattern of impulsivity and unstable relationships, affects, self-image, and behaviors, present by early adulthood and in a variety of contexts.
- At least five of the following must be present:
  1. Frantic efforts to avoid real or imagined abandonment.
  2. Unstable, intense interpersonal relationships (e.g., extreme love–hate relationships).
  3. Unstable self-image.
  4. Impulsivity in at least two potentially harmful ways (spending, sexual activity, substance use, binge eating, etc.).
  5. Recurrent suicidal threats or attempts or self-mutilation.
  6. Unstable mood/affect.
  7. Chronic feelings of emptiness.

8. Difficulty controlling anger.
9. Transient, stress-related paranoid ideation or dissociative symptoms.

Epidemiology
- Lifetime prevalence: Up to 6%.
- Diagnosed three times more often in women than men.
- Suicide rate: 10%.

Differential Diagnosis
- *Schizophrenia:* Unlike patients with schizophrenia, patients with BPD do not have frank psychosis (may have transient psychosis, however, if they decompensate under stress or substances of abuse).
- *Bipolar I/II:* Mood swings experienced in BPD are rapid, brief, moment-to-moment reactions to perceived environmental or psychological triggers.

Course
- Variable, but many develop stability in middle age.
- High incidence of coexisting major depression and/or substance use disorders.
- Increased risk of suicide.

Treatment
- Dialectical behavior therapy (DBT) is the treatment of choice—includes cognitive-behavioral therapy, mindfulness skills, and group therapy.
- Other psychotherapies found to be beneficial include mentalization-based therapy, transference-focused therapy, and schema-focused therapy.
- Pharmacotherapy should be considered an adjunct to psychotherapy. Various medications (e.g., mood stabilizers, antipsychotics, antidepressants) have been found to be somewhat effective in treating certain symptoms of BPD.

WARDS TIP

Borderline patients commonly use the defense mechanism of *splitting*—they view others and themselves as all good or all bad. (Clinical example: "You are the only doctor who has ever helped me. Every doctor I met before you was horrible.")

WARDS TIP

Pharmacotherapy has been shown to be more useful in BPD than in any other personality disorder.

HISTRIONIC PERSONALITY DISORDER (HPD)

Patients with histrionic personality disorder (HPD) exhibit attention-seeking behavior and excessive emotionality. They are dramatic, flamboyant, and extroverted, but are unable to form long-lasting, meaningful relationships. They are often sexually inappropriate and provocative.

Diagnosis and DSM-5 Criteria
- Pattern of excessive emotionality and attention seeking, present by early adulthood and in a variety of contexts.
- At least five of the following must be present:
  1. Uncomfortable when not the center of attention.
  2. Inappropriately seductive or provocative behavior.
  3. Rapidly shifting but shallow expression of emotion.
  4. Uses physical appearance to draw attention to self.
  5. Speech that is impressionistic and lacking in detail.
  6. Theatrical and exaggerated expression of emotion.
  7. Easily influenced by others or situation.
  8. Perceives relationships as more intimate than they actually are.

Epidemiology
- Prevalence: 2%.
- Women are more likely to have HPD than men.

Differential Diagnosis

Borderline personality disorder: Patients with BPD are more likely to suffer from depression, brief psychotic episodes, and to attempt suicide. HPD patients are generally more functional.

Course

Usually chronic, with some improvement of symptoms with age.

Treatment

- Psychotherapy (e.g., supportive, problem-solving, interpersonal, group) is the treatment of choice.
- Pharmacotherapy to treat associated depressive or anxious symptoms as necessary.

WARDS TIP

Histrionic patients often use the defense mechanism of *regression*—they revert to childlike behaviors.

NARCISSISTIC PERSONALITY DISORDER (NPD)

Patients with narcissistic personality disorder (NPD) have a sense of superiority, a need for admiration, and a lack of empathy. They consider themselves "special" and will exploit others for their own gain. Despite their grandiosity, however, these patients often have fragile self-esteem.

Diagnosis and DSM-5 Criteria

- Pattern of grandiosity, need for admiration, and lack of empathy beginning by early adulthood and present in a variety of contexts.
- Five or more of the following must be present:
  1. Exaggerated sense of self-importance.
  2. Preoccupation with fantasies of unlimited money, success, brilliance, etc.
  3. Believes that he or she is "special" or unique and can associate only with other high-status individuals.
  4. Requires excessive admiration.
  5. Has sense of entitlement.
  6. Takes advantage of others for self-gain.
  7. Lacks empathy.
  8. Envious of others or believes others are envious of him or her.
  9. Arrogant or haughty.

Epidemiology

Prevalence: Up to 6%.

Differential Diagnosis

Antisocial personality disorder: Both types of patients exploit others, but NPD patients want status and recognition, while antisocial patients want material gain or simply the subjugation of others. Narcissistic patients become depressed when they don't get the recognition they think they deserve.

Course

Usually has a chronic course; higher incidence of depression and midlife crises since these patients put such a high value on youth and power.

WARDS TIP

Narcissism is characterized by an inflated sense of entitlement. People with narcissistic personality are often "fishing for compliments" and become irritated and anxious when they are not treated as important.

Treatment
- Psychotherapy is the treatment of choice.
- Psychotropics may be used if a comorbid psychiatric disorder is also diagnosed.

Cluster C

Includes avoidant, dependent, and obsessive-compulsive personality disorders. These patients appear anxious and fearful (see Table 6-3).

AVOIDANT PERSONALITY DISORDER

Patients with avoidant personality disorder have a pervasive pattern of social inhibition and an intense fear of rejection. They will avoid situations in which they may be rejected. Their fear of rejection is so overwhelming that it affects all aspects of their lives. They avoid social interactions and may seek jobs in which there is little interpersonal contact. These patients *desire* companionship but are extremely shy and easily injured.

Diagnosis and DSM-5 Criteria
- A pattern of social inhibition, hypersensitivity, and feelings of inadequacy since early adulthood.
- At least four of the following must be present:
  1. Avoids occupation that involves interpersonal contact due to a fear of criticism and rejection.
  2. Unwilling to interact unless certain of being liked.
  3. Cautious of interpersonal relationships.
  4. Preoccupied with being criticized or rejected in social situations.
  5. Inhibited in new social situations because he or she feels inadequate.
  6. Believes he or she is socially inept and inferior.
  7. Reluctant to engage in new activities for fear of embarrassment.

KEY FACT

Avoidant personality disorder has large overlap with social anxiety disorder (social phobia); may be same syndrome/spectrum.

WARDS TIP

Symptoms of avoidant personality disorder—
AFRAID
Avoids occupation with others
Fear of embarrassment and criticism
Reserved unless they are certain that they are liked
Always thinking rejection
Isolates from relationships
Distances self unless certain that they are liked

TABLE 6-3. Cluster C Personality Disorders and Classic Clinical Examples

Personality Disorder	Clinical Example
Avoidant personality disorder	A 30-year-old postal worker rarely goes out with her coworkers and often makes excuses when they ask her to join them because she is afraid they will not like her. She wishes to go out and meet new people but, according to her, she is too "shy."
Dependent personality disorder	A 40-year-old man who lives with his parents has trouble deciding how to get his car fixed. He calls his father at work several times to ask very trivial things. He has been unemployed over the past 3 years.
Obsessive-compulsive personality disorder	A 40-year-old secretary has been recently fired because of her inability to prepare some work projects in time. According to her, they were not in the right format and she had to revise them six times, which led to the delay. This has happened before but she feels that she is not given enough time.

Epidemiology
- Prevalence: 2.4%.
- Equally frequent in males and females.

Differential Diagnosis
- *Schizoid personality disorder:* Patients with avoidant personality disorder desire companionship but are extremely shy, whereas patients with schizoid personality disorder have little or no desire for companionship.
- *Social anxiety disorder (social phobia):* See Chap. 5, "Anxiety Disorders." Both involve fear and avoidance of social situations. If the symptoms are an integral part of the patient's personality and have been evident since adolescence, personality disorder is the more likely diagnosis. Social anxiety disorder involves a fear of *embarrassment* in a particular setting (speaking in public, urinating in public, etc.), whereas avoidant personality disorder is an overall fear of *rejection* and a sense of inadequacy. However, a patient can have both disorders concurrently and should carry both diagnoses if criteria for each are met.
- *Dependent personality disorder:* Avoidant personality disorder patients cling to relationships, similar to dependent personality disorder patients; however, avoidant patients are slow to get involved, whereas dependent patients actively and aggressively seek relationships.

Course
- Course is usually chronic, although may remit with age.
- Particularly difficult during adolescence, when attractiveness and socialization are important.
- Increased incidence of associated anxiety and depressive disorders.
- If support system fails, patient is left very susceptible to depression, anxiety, and anger.

> **KEY FACT**
>
> Schizoid patients *prefer* to be alone. Avoidant patients want to be with others but are too scared of rejection.

Treatment
- Psychotherapy, including assertiveness and social skills training, is most effective.
- Group therapy may also be beneficial.
- Selective serotonin reuptake inhibitors (SSRIs) may be prescribed for comorbid social anxiety disorder or major depression.

DEPENDENT PERSONALITY DISORDER (DPD)

Patients with dependent personality disorder (DPD) have poor self-confidence and fear of separation. They have an excessive need to be taken care of and allow others to make decisions for them. They feel helpless when left alone.

Diagnosis and DSM-5 Criteria
- A pattern of excessive need to be taken care of that leads to submissive and clinging behavior.
- At least five of the following must be present:
  1. Difficulty making everyday decisions without reassurance from others.
  2. Needs others to assume responsibilities for most areas of his or her life.
  3. Difficulty expressing disagreement because of fear of loss of approval.
  4. Difficulty initiating projects because of lack of self-confidence.
  5. Goes to excessive lengths to obtain support from others.
  6. Feels helpless when alone.

> **WARDS TIP**
>
> Symptoms of dependent personality disorder—
> **OBEDIENT**
> **O**bsessive about approval
> **B**ound by other's decisions
> **E**nterprises are rarely initiated due to their lack of self-confidence
> **D**ifficult to make own decisions
> **I**nvalid feelings while alone
> **E**ngrossed with fears of self-reliance
> **N**eeds to be in a relationship
> **T**entative about decisions

7. Urgently seeks another relationship when one ends.
8. Preoccupied with fears of being left to take care of self.

Epidemiology
- Prevalence: Approximately <1%.
- Women are more likely to be diagnosed with DPD than men.
- Childhood medical illness or separation anxiety disorder may increase the likelihood of developing DPD.

Differential Diagnosis
- *Avoidant personality disorder:* See discussion above.
- *Borderline and histrionic personality disorders:* Patients with DPD usually have a long-lasting relationship with one person on whom they are dependent. Patients with borderline and histrionic personality disorders are often dependent on other people, but they are unable to maintain a long-lasting relationship.

Course
- Usually has a chronic course.
- Patients are prone to depression, particularly after loss of person on whom they are dependent.
- Difficulties with employment since they cannot act independently or without close supervision.

Treatment
- Psychotherapy, particularly cognitive-behavioral, assertiveness, and social skills training, is the treatment of choice.
- Pharmacotherapy may be used to treat associated symptoms of anxiety or depression.

KEY FACT

Regression is often seen in people with DPD. This is defined as going back to a younger age of maturity.

WARDS TIP

Many people with debilitating illnesses can develop dependent traits. However, to be diagnosed with DPD, the features must manifest by early adulthood.

OBSESSIVE-COMPULSIVE PERSONALITY DISORDER (OCPD)

Patients with obssesive-compulsive personality disorder (OCPD) have a pervasive pattern of perfectionism, inflexibility, and orderliness. They become so preoccupied with unimportant details that they are often unable to complete simple tasks in a timely fashion. They appear stiff, serious, and formal, with constricted affect. They are often successful professionally but have poor interpersonal skills.

Diagnosis and DSM-5 Criteria
- Pattern of preoccupation with orderliness, control, and perfectionism at the expense of efficiency and flexibility, present by early adulthood and in a variety of contexts.
- At least four of the following must be present:
  1. Preoccupation with details, rules, lists, and organization such that the major point of the activity is lost.
  2. Perfectionism that is detrimental to completion of task.
  3. Excessive devotion to work.
  4. Excessive conscientiousness and scrupulousness about morals and ethics.
  5. Will not delegate tasks.
  6. Unable to discard worthless objects.
  7. Miserly spending style.
  8. Rigid and stubborn.

Epidemiology
- Prevalence: 2–7%.
- Men are two times more likely to have OCPD than women.

Differential Diagnosis
- *Obsessive-compulsive disorder (OCD):* Patients with OCPD do not have the recurrent obsessions or compulsions that are present in OCD. In addition, the symptoms of OCPD are **ego-syntonic** rather than ego-dystonic (as in OCD); OCD patients are aware that they have a problem and wish that their thoughts and behaviors would go away.
- *Narcissistic personality disorder:* Both personalities involve assertiveness and achievement, but NPD patients are motivated by status, whereas OCPD patients are motivated by the work itself.

Course
- Unpredictable course.
- Some patients can have comorbid OCD (most do not).

Treatment
- Psychotherapy is the treatment of choice. Cognitive-behavior therapy may be particularly useful.
- Pharmacotherapy may be used to treat associated symptoms as necessary.

PERSONALITY CHANGE DUE TO ANOTHER MEDICAL CONDITION

This refers to a persistent personality change from a previous pattern due to the direct pathophysiological result of a medical condition (e.g., head trauma, strokes, epilepsy, central nervous system infections, or neoplasms). Subtypes include labile, disinhibited, aggressive, apathetic, or paranoid.

OTHER SPECIFIED PERSONALITY DISORDER

This diagnosis is reserved for a personality disorder that does not meet the full criteria for any of the disorders, but where the clinician *chooses* to communicate the specific reason that the presentation does not meet the criteria for any specific personality disorder (e.g., "mixed personality disorder").

UNSPECIFIED PERSONALITY DISORDER

This diagnosis is used for a personality disorder that does not meet the full criteria for any of the disorders, but where the clinician chooses *not* to specify the reason that the criteria are not met for any specific personality disorder (e.g., not enough information to make a more specific diagnosis).

NOTES

CHAPTER 7
SUBSTANCE-RELATED AND ADDICTIVE DISORDERS

Substance Use Disorders	80
Diagnosis and DSM-5 Criteria	80
Epidemiology	80
Psychiatric Symptoms	80
Acute Intoxication and Withdrawal	80
Detection of Substance Use	81
Treatment of Substance Use Disorders	81
Alcohol (EtOH)	82
Intoxication	82
Withdrawal	83
Alcohol Use Disorder	85
Cocaine	87
Intoxication	87
Cocaine Use Disorder	87
Withdrawal	88
Amphetamines	88
Intoxication	88
Phencyclidine (PCP)	88
Intoxication	89
Withdrawal	89
Sedative-Hypnotics	89
Intoxication	89
Withdrawal	90
Opioids	90
Intoxication	90
Opiate Use Disorder	91
Withdrawal	91
Hallucinogens	92
Intoxication	92
Withdrawal	92
Marijuana	92
Intoxication	92
Withdrawal	93
Inhalants	93
Intoxication	93
Withdrawal	93
Caffeine	94
Overdose	94
Withdrawal	94
Nicotine	94
Treatment of Nicotine Dependence	94
Gambling Disorder	95
Diagnosis and DSM-5 Criteria	95
Epidemiology/Etiology	95
Treatment	95

Substance Use Disorders

Substance use disorders are characterized by a problematic pattern of substance use that leads to some form of functional impairment or distress. Keep in mind that frequent use of a substance does not necessarily indicate a *substance use disorder* unless it is causing problems for the patient.

DIAGNOSIS AND DSM-5 CRITERIA

Substance use disorders are characterized by a problematic pattern of substance use causing impairment or distress, as manifested by at least two of the following within a 12-month period:

- Using substance more than originally intended.
- Persistent desire or unsuccessful efforts to cut down on use.
- Significant time spent in obtaining, using, or recovering from substance.
- Craving to use substance.
- Failure to fulfill obligations at work, school, or home.
- Continued use despite social or interpersonal problems due to the substance use.
- Limiting social, occupational, or recreational activities because of substance use.
- Use in dangerous situations (e.g., driving a car).
- Continued use despite subsequent physical or psychological problem (e.g., drinking alcohol despite worsening liver problems).
- Tolerance (needing higher amounts of the substance to achieve the desired effect *or* experiencing diminished effects when repeating the same dose).
- Withdrawal (a substance-specific syndrome occurring when a patient stops or reduces heavy/prolonged substance use).

Note that these criteria remain the same regardless of what substance(s) the patient is using.

EPIDEMIOLOGY

- One-year prevalence of any substance use disorder in the United States is approximately 8%.
- More common in men than women.
- Alcohol and nicotine are the most commonly used substances.

PSYCHIATRIC SYMPTOMS

- Mood symptoms are common among persons with substance use disorders.
- Psychotic symptoms may occur with some substances.
- Personality disorders and psychiatric comorbidities (e.g., major depression, anxiety disorders) are common among persons with substance use disorders.
- It is often challenging to decide whether psychiatric symptoms are primary or substance-induced.

ACUTE INTOXICATION AND WITHDRAWAL

Both the intoxicated and withdrawing patient can present difficulties in diagnosis and treatment. Since it is common for persons to abuse several

WARDS TIP

It is possible to have a substance use disorder without having physiological dependence (i.e., without having withdrawal or tolerance).

WARDS TIP

Substance-induced mood symptoms improve during prolonged abstinence, whereas *primary* mood symptoms persist.

KEY FACT

Withdrawal symptoms of a drug are usually the opposite of its intoxication effects. For example, alcohol is sedating, but alcohol *withdrawal* can cause brain excitation and seizures.

TABLE 7-1. Direct Testing for Substance Use

Substance	Details
Alcohol	■ Stays in system for only a few hours. ■ Breathalyzer test, commonly used by law enforcement. ■ Blood/urine testing more accurate.
Cocaine	■ Urine drug screen positive for 2–4 days.
Amphetamines	■ Urine drug screen positive for 1–3 days. ■ Most assays have poor sensitivity and/or specificity.
Phencyclidine (PCP)	■ Urine drug screen positive for 4–7 days. ■ Creatine kinase (CK) and aspartate aminotransferase (AST) are often elevated.
Sedative-hypnotics	In urine and blood for variable amounts of time. *Barbiturates:* ■ Short-acting (pentobarbital): 24 hours ■ Long-acting (phenobarbital): 3 weeks *Benzodiazepines:* ■ Short-acting (e.g., lorazepam): up to 5 days ■ Long-acting (diazepam): up to 30 days
Opioids	■ Urine drug test remains positive for 1–3 days, depending on opioid used. ■ Methadone and oxycodone will come up negative on a general screen (order a separate panel).
Marijuana	Urine detection: ■ After a single use, about 3 days. In heavy users, up to 4 weeks (THC is released from adipose stores).

KEY FACT

Pregnant women should not drink alcohol as it can increase fetal alcohol syndrome in the newborn, which is a potential cause of intellectual disability.

substances at once, the clinical presentation is often confusing, and signs/symptoms may be atypical. Always be on the lookout for use of multiple substances.

DETECTION OF SUBSTANCE USE

See Table 7-1.

TREATMENT OF SUBSTANCE USE DISORDERS

- Behavioral counseling should be part of every substance use disorder treatment.
- Psychosocial treatments are effective and include motivational intervention (MI), cognitive-behavioral therapy (CBT), contingency management, and individual and group therapy.
- Twelve-step groups such as Alcoholics Anonymous (AA) and Narcotics Anonymous (NA) should also be encouraged as part of the treatment.
- Pharmacotherapy is available for some drugs of abuse, and will be discussed later in this chapter as relevant to a particular substance.

Alcohol (EtOH)

- Alcohol activates gamma-aminobutyric acid (GABA), dopamine, and serotonin receptors in the central nervous system (CNS). It inhibits glutamate receptor activity and voltage-gated calcium channels. GABA receptors are inhibitory, and glutamate receptors are excitatory; thus, alcohol is a potent CNS depressant.
- Lifetime prevalence of alcohol use disorder in the United States is 5% of women and 12% of men.
- Alcohol is metabolized in the following manner:
  1. Alcohol → acetaldehyde (enzyme: *alcohol dehydrogenase*).
  2. Acetaldehyde → acetic acid (enzyme: *aldehyde dehydrogenase*).

These enzymes are upregulated in heavy drinkers. Secondary to a gene variant, Asians often have less aldehyde dehydrogenase, resulting in flushing and nausea with alcohol use.

INTOXICATION

Clinical Presentation

- The absorption and elimination rates of alcohol are variable and depend on many factors, including age, sex, body weight, chronic nature of use, duration of consumption, food in the stomach, and the state of nutrition and liver health.
- In addition to the above factors, the effects of EtOH also depend on the blood alcohol level (BAL). Serum EtOH level or an expired air breathalyzer can determine the extent of intoxication. As shown in Table 7-2, patients with high tolerance may show diminished effects at a given BAL.

Treatment

- **Monitor:** Airway, breathing, circulation, glucose, electrolytes, acid–base status.
- Give parenteral **thiamine** (to prevent or treat Wernicke's encephalopathy) and folate. Remember thiamine must be given before glucose, as it's a necessary cofactor for glucose metabolism.
- **Naloxone** may be necessary to reverse effects of co-ingested opioids.

> **WARDS TIP**
>
> Alcohol is the most common co-ingestant in drug overdoses.

> **KEY FACT**
>
> Most adults will show some signs of intoxication with BAL > 100 and obvious signs with BAL > 150 mg/dL.

> **KEY FACT**
>
> Ethanol, along with methanol and ethylene glycol, can be a cause of anion gap metabolic acidosis.

TABLE 7-2. Clinical Presentation of Alcohol Intoxication

Effects	BAL
Impaired fine motor control	20–50 mg/dL
Impaired judgment and coordination	50–100 mg/dL
Ataxic gait and poor balance	100–150 mg/dL
Lethargy, difficulty sitting upright, difficulty with memory, nausea/vomiting	150–250 mg/dL
Coma (in the novice drinker)	300 mg/dL
Respiratory depression, death possible	400 mg/dL

- A computed tomography (CT) scan of the head may be necessary to rule out subdural hematoma or other brain injury.
- The liver will eventually metabolize alcohol without any other interventions.
- Severely intoxicated patients may require mechanical ventilation with attention to acid–base balance, temperature, and electrolytes while they are recovering.
- Gastrointestinal evacuation (e.g., gastric lavage, induction of emesis, and charcoal) is not indicated in the treatment of EtOH overdose unless a significant amount of EtOH was ingested within the preceding 30–60 minutes.

WITHDRAWAL

 A 42-year-old man has routine surgery for a knee injury. After 72 hours in the hospital he becomes anxious, flushed, diaphoretic, hypertensive, and tachycardic. *What most likely accounts for this patient's symptoms?* Alcohol withdrawal. *Treatment?* Benzodiazepines (chlordiazepoxide [Librium] or lorazepam [Ativan] are considered the drugs of choice). *What are you most concerned about?* Seizures, delirium tremens, autonomic instability, and cardiac arrhythmias. Remember that alcohol withdrawal can be fatal.

> **KEY FACT**
>
> Males with substance use disorders, especially alcohol, have higher rates of perpetrating domestic violence.

> **KEY FACT**
>
> Alcohol is the most commonly used intoxicating substance in the United States.

Chronic alcohol use has a depressant effect on the CNS, and cessation of use causes a compensatory hyperactivity with glutamate excitotoxicity. Alcohol withdrawal is **potentially lethal!**

Clinical Presentation

- Signs and symptoms of **alcohol withdrawal syndrome** include insomnia, anxiety, hand tremor, irritability, anorexia, nausea, vomiting, autonomic hyperactivity (diaphoresis, tachycardia, hypertension), psychomotor agitation, fever, seizures, hallucinations, and delirium tremens (see Table 7-3).
- The earliest symptoms of EtOH withdrawal begin between 6 and 24 hours after the patient's last drink and depend on the duration and quantity of EtOH consumption, liver size, and body mass.
- Generalized tonic-clonic seizures usually occur between 12 and 48 hours after cessation of drinking, with a peak around 12–24 hours.
- About a third of persons with seizures develop delirium tremens (DTs).
- Hypomagnesemia may predispose to seizures; thus, it should be corrected promptly.
- Seizures are treated with benzodiazepines. Long-term treatment with anticonvulsants is not recommended for alcohol withdrawal seizures.

TABLE 7-3. Alcohol Withdrawal Symptoms

Alcohol withdrawal symptoms usually begin in 6–24 hours after the last drink and may last 2–7 days.
Mild: Irritability, tremor, insomnia.
Moderate: Diaphoresis, hypertension, tachycardia, fever, disorientation.
Severe: Tonic-clonic seizures, DTs, hallucinations.

KEY FACT

Risk of suicide attempts is higher among those with psychiatric disorders and substance use (especially alcohol).

KEY FACT

Delirium tremens is a dangerous form of alcohol withdrawal involving mental status and neurological changes. Symptoms include disorientation, agitation, visual and tactile hallucinations, and autonomic instability (increase in respiratory rate, heart rate, and blood pressure). It carries a 5% mortality rate but occurs in only 5% of patients that experience EtOH withdrawal. Treatment includes supportive care and benzodiazepines.

KEY FACT

Confabulation—inventing stories of events that never occurred—is often associated with Korsakoff's "psychosis," or alcohol-induced neurocognitive disorder. Patients are unaware that they are "making things up."

Delirium Tremens

- The most serious form of EtOH withdrawal.
- Usually begins 48–96 hours after the last drink but may occur later.
- While only 5% of patients who experience EtOH withdrawal develop DTs, there is a roughly 5% mortality rate (up to 35% if left untreated).
- Physical illness predisposes to the condition.
- Age >30 and prior DTs increase the risk.
- In addition to delirium, symptoms of DTs may include hallucinations (most commonly visual), agitation, gross tremor, autonomic instability, and fluctuating levels of psychomotor activity.
- It is a medical emergency and should be treated with adequate doses of benzodiazepines.

Treatment

- Benzodiazepines (lorazepam, diazepam, or chlordiazepoxide) should be given in sufficient doses to keep the patient calm and lightly sedated, then tapered down slowly. Carbamazepine or valproic acid can be used in mild withdrawal.
- Thiamine, folic acid, and a multivitamin to treat nutritional deficiencies ("banana bag").
- Electrolyte and fluid abnormalities must be corrected.
- Monitor withdrawal signs and symptoms with the Clinical Institute Withdrawal Assessment (CIWA) scale.
- Providers must pay careful attention to the level of consciousness, and consider the possibility of traumatic injuries.
- Check for signs of hepatic failure (e.g., ascites, jaundice, caput medusae, coagulopathy).

Alcoholic ketoacidosis

- Frequently seen in the setting of alcohol cessation after an alcohol binge secondary to protracted vomiting and lack of oral intake.
- Hallmark is ketosis without hyperglycemia and a negative alcohol level.
- Laboratory studies reveal a high anion gap metabolic acidosis, ketonemia, and low levels of potassium, magnesium, and phosphorus.
- Treatment consists of hydration with D5NS, and replacing electrolytes.

Mr. Smith is a 42-year-old divorced man who arrives to the ED requesting treatment for alcohol detoxification. He began drinking at the age of 17. Although he initially drank only on the weekends, his alcohol use gradually progressed to drinking half a pint of whiskey daily by the age of 35. At that time, he arrived to his workplace intoxicated on several occasions and was referred to a 45-day inpatient alcohol addiction program. After completing the program, he was able to maintain sobriety for 7 years. However, 2 years ago he got divorced, was laid off from work, and ultimately relapsed into alcohol use.

Mr. Smith is currently living with his older sister and states that his drinking is "out of control." He had a DUI recently and has a court date in 2 weeks. He has tried to quit alcohol on his own on several occasions. However, when he stops drinking he feels "shaky, sweaty, anxious, and irritable" and thus resumes his alcohol intake. He also reports a history of a seizure 10 years ago, after he abruptly discontinued his alcohol use for a few days.

Mr. Smith's last drink was about 8 hours prior to his arrival at the ED. During the last month he has been feeling sad, with low energy, difficulty falling and staying asleep, low appetite, and difficulty concentrating. He denies suicidal ideation but has significant guilt over not being able to stop drinking. He denies a history of depression or anxiety, and has not received any other psychiatric treatment in the past.

Upon presentation to ER the patient's blood alcohol level was 110, he did not have symptoms of intoxication, and his urine drug screen was negative. Vital signs were significant for blood pressure of 150/90 and pulse of 110 bpm. Complete blood count and electrolytes were within normal limits.

What is Mr. Smith's most likely diagnosis?

The patient has a diagnosis of alcohol use disorder, with current signs of withdrawal. It is clear that he has exhibited symptoms of tolerance and withdrawal, has been using more alcohol than intended, and has made unsuccessful efforts to cut down. He also describes symptoms suggestive of a depressive disorder. The fact that his depressive symptoms began while abusing alcohol warrants a diagnosis of alcohol-induced depressive disorder. However, major depressive disorder should be ruled out once he remits his alcohol use. If his depressive symptoms are indeed substance-induced, they will improve and resolve with continuing sobriety.

What would be the next step in management?

Given the Mr. Smith's heavy chronic alcohol use and history of complicated withdrawal (i.e., seizure), he should be admitted to an inpatient unit for close monitoring. Outpatient detoxification is not appropriate in this case. He will likely require a standing and PRN benzodiazepine (the particular benzodiazepine sometimes varies depending on hospital's protocol), as well as close monitoring for signs of withdrawal.

ALCOHOL USE DISORDER

- The **AUDIT-C** (Table 7-4) is used to screen for alcohol use disorder.
- Biochemical markers are useful in detecting recent prolonged drinking; ongoing monitoring of biomarkers can also help detect a relapse. Most commonly used biomarkers are BAL, liver function tests (LFTs—aspartate aminotransferase [AST], alanine aminotransferase [ALT]), gamma-glutamyl transpeptidase (GGT), and mean corpuscular volume (MCV).

Medications for Alcohol Use Disorder

First-line treatments:
- Naltrexone (Revia, IM-Vivitrol): *Cannot be given if LFTs are elevated*
    - Opioid receptor antagonist.
    - Reduces desire/craving and the "high" associated with alcohol.
    - May see greater benefit in men with a family history of alcoholism.
    - Will precipitate withdrawal in patients with physical opioid dependence.
- Acamprosate (Campral):
    - Thought to modulate glutamate transmission. *Pt needs to abstain from EtOH before starting acamprosate.*

WARDS TIP

At-risk or heavy drinking for men is more than 4 drinks per day or more than 14 drinks per week. For women, it is more than 3 drinks per day or more than 7 drinks per week.

TABLE 7-4. AUDIT-C

QUESTION #1: HOW OFTEN DID YOU HAVE A DRINK CONTAINING ALCOHOL IN THE PAST YEAR?

■ Never	(0 points)
■ Monthly or less	(1 point)
■ Two to four times a month	(2 points)
■ Two to three times per week	(3 points)
■ Four or more times a week	(4 points)

QUESTION #2: HOW MANY DRINKS DID YOU HAVE ON A TYPICAL DAY WHEN YOU WERE DRINKING IN THE PAST YEAR?

■ 1 or 2	(0 points)
■ 3 or 4	(1 point)
■ 5 or 6	(2 points)
■ 7 to 9	(3 points)
■ 10 or more	(4 points)

QUESTION #3: HOW OFTEN DID YOU HAVE SIX OR MORE DRINKS ON ONE OCCASION IN THE PAST YEAR?

■ Never	(0 points)
■ Less than monthly	(1 point)
■ Monthly	(2 points)
■ Weekly	(3 points)
■ Daily or almost daily	(4 points)

The AUDIT-C is scored on a scale of 0–12 (scores of 0 reflect no alcohol use). In men, a score of 4 or more is considered positive; in women, a score of 3 or more is considered positive.

- Use for relapse prevention in patients who have stopped drinking (post-detoxification).
- Major advantage is that it can be used in patients with liver disease.
- Contraindicated in severe renal disease.

Second-line treatments:
- Disulfiram (Antabuse):
  - Blocks the enzyme aldehyde dehydrogenase in the liver, causing aversive reactions to alcohol (flushing, headache, nausea/vomiting, palpitations, shortness of breath).
  - Contraindicated in severe cardiac disease, pregnancy, and psychosis.
  - Liver function should be monitored.
  - Best used in highly motivated patients, as medication adherence is an issue.

- Topiramate (Topamax):
  - Anticonvulsant that potentiates GABA and inhibits glutamate receptors.
  - Reduces cravings for alcohol and decreases alcohol use.

Long-Term Complications of Alcohol Intake
- **Wernicke's encephalopathy:**
  - Caused by thiamine (vitamin B_1) deficiency resulting from poor nutrition.
  - Acute and can be reversed with thiamine therapy.
  - Features: Ataxia (broad-based), confusion, ocular abnormalities (nystagmus, gaze palsies).
- If left untreated, Wernicke's encephalopathy may progress to **Korsakoff syndrome:**
  - Chronic amnestic syndrome.
  - Reversible in only about 20% of patients.
  - Features: Impaired recent memory, anterograde amnesia, compensatory confabulation (unconsciously making up answers when memory has failed).

Cocaine

Cocaine blocks the reuptake of dopamine, epinephrine, and norepinephrine from the synaptic cleft, causing a stimulant effect. Dopamine plays a role in the behavioral reinforcement ("reward") system of the brain.

INTOXICATION
- *General:* Euphoria, heightened self-esteem, increase or decrease in blood pressure, tachycardia or bradycardia, nausea, dilated pupils, weight loss, psychomotor agitation or depression, chills, and sweating.
- *Dangerous:* Seizures, cardiac arrhythmias, hyperthermia, paranoia, and hallucinations (especially tactile). Since cocaine is an indirect sympathomimetic, intoxication mimics the fight-or-flight response.
- *Deadly:* Cocaine's vasoconstrictive effect may result in myocardial infarction (MI), intracranial hemorrhage, or stroke.

Management
- For mild-to-moderate agitation and anxiety: Reassurance of the patient and benzodiazepines.
- For severe agitation or psychosis: Antipsychotics (e.g., haloperidol).
- Symptomatic support (i.e., control hypertension, arrhythmias).
- Temperature of >102°F should be treated aggressively with an ice bath, cooling blanket, **and other supportive measures.**

COCAINE USE DISORDER

Treatment of cocaine use disorder
- There is no Food and Drug Administration (FDA)-approved pharmacotherapy for cocaine use disorder.
- Off-label medications are sometimes used (naltrexone, modafinil, topiramate).
- Psychological interventions (contingency management, relapse prevention, NA, etc.) are the mainstay of treatment.

KEY FACT

AST:ALT ratio ≥2:1 and elevated GGT suggest excessive long-term alcohol use; they take a few weeks to return to normal during abstinence.

KEY FACT

Alcohol can cause increase in LFTs and macrocytosis (increase in MCV).

WARDS TIP

Give all patients with altered mental status thiamine *before* glucose, to avoid precipitating Wernicke–Korsakoff syndrome. Thiamine is a coenzyme used in carbohydrate metabolism.

KEY FACT

Cocaine overdose can cause death secondary to cardiac arrhythmia, MI, seizure, or respiratory depression.

WITHDRAWAL

- Abrupt abstinence is not life threatening.
- Produces post-intoxication depression ("crash"): Malaise, fatigue, hypersomnolence, depression, anhedonia, hunger, constricted pupils, vivid dreams, psychomotor agitation, or retardation. Occasionally, these patients can become suicidal.
- With mild-to-moderate cocaine use, withdrawal symptoms resolve within 72 hours; with heavy, chronic use, they may last for 1–2 weeks.
- Treatment is supportive, but severe psychiatric symptoms may warrant hospitalization.

Amphetamines

KEY FACT

Heavy amphetamine use may induce psychosis, mimicking schizophrenia.

- Classic amphetamines:
  - Block reuptake and facilitate release of dopamine and norepinephrine from nerve endings, causing a stimulant effect.
  - *Examples:* Dextroamphetamine (Dexedrine), methylphenidate (Ritalin), methamphetamine (Desoxyn, "ice," "speed," "crystal meth," "crank").
  - Methamphetamines are easily manufactured in home laboratories using over-the-counter medications (e.g., pseudoephedrine).
  - Methamphetamines are used medically in the treatment of narcolepsy, attention deficit/hyperactivity disorder (ADHD), binge eating, and occasionally depressive disorders.
- Substituted ("designer," "club drugs") amphetamines:
  - Release dopamine, norepinephrine, and serotonin from nerve endings.
  - *Examples:* MDMA ("ecstasy"), MDEA ("eve").
  - Often used in dance clubs and raves.
  - Have both stimulant and hallucinogenic properties.
  - Serotonin syndrome is possible if designer amphetamines are combined with selective serotonin reuptake inhibitors (SSRIs).

KEY FACT

Symptoms of amphetamine intoxication include euphoria, dilated pupils, increased libido, tachycardia, perspiration, grinding teeth, and chest pain.

INTOXICATION

Clinical Presentation

- Amphetamine intoxication causes symptoms similar to those of cocaine (see above).
- MDMA and MDEA may induce sense of closeness to others.
- Overdose can cause hyperthermia, dehydration (especially after a prolonged period of dancing in a club), rhabdomyolysis, and renal failure.
- Complications of their long half-life can cause ongoing psychosis, even during abstinence.
- Amphetamine withdrawal can cause prolonged depression.

WARDS TIP

Chronic amphetamine use leads to accelerated tooth decay ("meth mouth").

Treatment

Rehydrate, correct electrolyte balance, and treat hyperthermia.

Phencyclidine (PCP)

WARDS TIP

Both amphetamine and PCP use can cause rhabdomyolysis. Look for elevated creatine kinase (CK) and monitor closely for acute kidney injury. Treatment is mostly supportive and emphasizes hydration.

PCP, or "angel dust," is a dissociative, hallucinogenic drug that antagonizes *N*-methyl-D-aspartate (NMDA) glutamate receptors and activates dopaminergic neurons. It can have stimulant or CNS depressant effects, depending on the dose taken.

- PCP can be smoked as "wet" (sprinkled on cigarette) or as a "joint" (sprinkled on marijuana).
- Ketamine is similar to PCP, but is less potent. Ketamine is sometimes used as a "date rape" drug, as it is odorless and tasteless.

INTOXICATION

Clinical Presentation
- Effects include agitation, depersonalization, hallucinations, synesthesia (one sensory stimulation evokes another—e.g., hearing a sound causes one to see a color), impaired judgment, memory impairment, combativeness, **nystagmus** (rotary, horizontal, or vertical), ataxia, dysarthria, hypertension, tachycardia, muscle rigidity, and high tolerance to pain.
- Overdose can cause seizures, delirium, coma, and even death.

Treatment
- Monitor vitals, temperature, and electrolytes, and minimize sensory stimulation.
- Use benzodiazepines (lorazepam) to treat agitation, anxiety, muscle spasms, and seizures.
- Use antipsychotics (haloperidol) to control severe agitation or psychotic symptoms.

WITHDRAWAL

No withdrawal syndrome, but "flashbacks" (recurrence of intoxication symptoms due to release of the drug from body lipid stores) may occur.

Sedative-Hypnotics

Agents in the sedative-hypnotics category include benzodiazepines, barbiturates, zolpidem, zaleplon, gamma-hydroxybutyrate (GHB), meprobamate, and others. These medications, especially benzodiazepines, are highly abused in the United States, as they are more readily available than other drugs such as cocaine.

- Benzodiazepines (BZDs):
  - Commonly used in the treatment of anxiety disorders.
  - Easily obtained via prescription from physicians' offices and emergency departments.
  - Potentiate the effects of GABA by modulating the receptor, thereby increasing frequency of chloride channel opening.
- Barbiturates:
  - Used in the treatment of epilepsy and as anesthetics.
  - Potentiate the effects of GABA by binding to the receptor and increasing duration of chloride channel opening.
  - At high doses, barbiturates act as direct GABA agonists, and therefore have a lower margin of safety relative to BZDs.
  - They are synergistic in combination with BZDs (as well as other CNS depressants such as alcohol); respiratory depression can occur.

INTOXICATION

Clinical Presentation
- Intoxication with sedatives produces drowsiness, confusion, hypotension, slurred speech, incoordination, ataxia, mood lability, impaired judgment, nystagmus, respiratory depression, and coma or death in overdose.

KEY FACT

Ketamine ("special K") can produce tachycardia, tachypnea, hallucinations, and amnesia.

KEY FACT

PCP intoxication symptoms—
RED DANES
Rage
Erythema (redness of skin)
Dilated pupils
Delusions
Amnesia
Nystagmus
Excitation
Skin dryness

KEY FACT

Rotatory nystagmus is pathognomonic of PCP intoxication.

KEY FACT

Tactile and visual hallucinations are found in both cocaine and PCP intoxication.

KEY FACT

PCP intoxication is associated with violence, more so than other drugs.

KEY FACT

Gamma-hydroxybutyrate (GHB) is a CNS depressant that produces confusion, dizziness, drowsiness, memory loss, respiratory distress, and coma. It is commonly used as a date-rape drug.

KEY FACT

Barbiturate withdrawal can be deadly, and has the highest mortality rate of all the kinds of substance withdrawals.

WARDS TIP

Flumazenil is a very short-acting BZD antagonist used for treating BZD overdose. Use with caution when treating overdose, as it may precipitate seizures.

KEY FACT

In general, withdrawal from drugs that are sedating (e.g., alcohol, barbiturates, benzodiazepines) is life threatening, while withdrawal from stimulants (e.g., cocaine, amphetamines) is not.

KEY FACT

The opioid dextromethorphan is a common ingredient in cough syrup.

KEY FACT

Infection secondary to needle sharing is a common cause of morbidity from street heroin usage.

- Symptoms are synergistic when combined with EtOH or opioids/narcotics.
- Long-term sedative use may lead to dependence and may cause depressive symptoms.

Treatment

- Maintain airway, breathing, and circulation. Monitor vital signs.
- Activated charcoal and gastric lavage to prevent further gastrointestinal absorption (if drug was ingested in the prior 4–6 hours).
- For *barbiturates only:* Alkalinize urine with sodium bicarbonate to promote renal excretion.
- For *benzodiazepines only:* Flumazenil in overdose.
- Supportive care—improve respiratory status, control hypotension.

WITHDRAWAL

Abrupt abstinence after chronic use can be **life threatening**. While physiological dependence is more likely with short-acting agents, longer-acting agents can also cause dependence and withdrawal symptoms.

Clinical Presentation

Signs and symptoms of withdrawal are the same as these of EtOH withdrawal. Tonic-clonic seizures may occur and can be life threatening.

Treatment

- Benzodiazepines (stabilize patient, then taper gradually).
- Carbamazepine or valproic acid taper not as beneficial.

Opioids

- Opioid medications and drugs of abuse stimulate mu, kappa, and delta opiate receptors (normally stimulated by endogenous opiates), and are involved in analgesia, sedation, and dependence. Examples include heroin, oxycodone, codeine, dextromethorphan, morphine, methadone, and meperidine (Demerol).
- Opioids also have effects on the dopaminergic system, which mediates their addictive and rewarding properties.
- Prescription opioids (OxyContin [oxycodone], Vicodin [hydrocodone/acetaminophen], and Percocet [oxycodone/acetaminophen])—not heroin—are the most commonly used opioids.
- Behaviors such as losing medication, "doctor shopping," and running out of medication early should alert clinicians of possible misuse.
- Opioids are associated with more deaths (usually due to unintentional overdose) than any other drug.

INTOXICATION

Clinical Presentation

- Opioid intoxication causes drowsiness, nausea/vomiting, constipation, slurred speech, **constricted pupils**, seizures, and respiratory depression, which may progress to coma or death in overdose.
- Meperidine and monoamine oxidase inhibitors taken in combination may cause **serotonin syndrome**: hyperthermia, confusion, hypertension or hypotension, and hyperreflexia.

Treatment

- Ensure adequate airway, breathing, and circulation.
- In overdose, administration of naloxone (an opioid antagonist) will improve respiratory depression but may cause severe withdrawal in an opioid-dependent patient.
- Ventilatory support may be required.
- Patients at risk of opioid overdose should be prescribed a naloxone (Narcan) kit to keep at home for emergencies.

OPIATE USE DISORDER

See Table 7-5 for treatment of opioid use disorder.

WITHDRAWAL

- While not life threatening, abstinence in the opioid-dependent individual leads to an unpleasant withdrawal syndrome characterized by dysphoria, insomnia, lacrimation, rhinorrhea, yawning, weakness, sweating,

TABLE 7-5. Pharmacological Treatment of Opioid Use Disorder

Medication	Mechanism	Pros	Cons
Methadone	Long-acting opioid receptor agonist	Administered once daily. Significantly reduces morbidity and mortality in opioid-dependent persons.	Restricted to federally licensed substance abuse treatment programs. Can cause QTc interval prolongation: screening electrocardiogram is indicated, particularly in patients with high risk of cardiac disease.
Buprenorphine	Partial opioid receptor agonist—can precipitate withdrawal if used too soon after full opioid agonists	Sublingual preparation that is safer than methadone, as its effects reach a plateau and make overdose unlikely. Comes as Suboxone, which contains buprenorphine and naloxone; this preparation prevents intoxication from intravenous injection.	Only available by prescription from specially licensed office-based physicians.
Naltrexone	Competitive opioid antagonist, precipitates withdrawal if used within 7 days of heroin use	Either daily oral medication or monthly depot injection. It is a good choice for highly motivated patients such as health care professionals.	Compliance is an issue for oral formulation.

KEY FACT

Opioid intoxication: nausea, vomiting, sedation, decrease in pain perception, decrease in gastrointestinal motility, pupil constriction, and respiratory depression (which *can be fatal*).

KEY FACT

Meperidine is the exception to opioids producing miosis. "Demerol Dilates pupils."

KEY FACT

Naloxone is the treatment of choice for opiate overdose.

WARDS TIP

Classic triad of opioid overdose—
Rebels **A**dmire **M**orphine
Respiratory depression
Altered mental status
Miosis

KEY FACT

Eating large amounts of poppy seed bagels or muffins can result in a urine drug screen that is positive for opioids.

WARDS TIP

Rapid recovery of consciousness following the administration of intravenous (IV) naloxone (a potent opioid antagonist) is consistent with opioid overdose.

KEY FACT

Remember the withdrawal symptoms of opiates: flu-like symptoms (body aches, anorexia, rhinorrhea, fever), diarrhea, anxiety, insomnia, and piloerection. These are *not* life threatening.

KEY FACT

An LSD flashback is a spontaneous recurrence of symptoms mimicking a prior LSD "trip" that may last for minutes to hours.

piloerection, nausea/vomiting, fever, dilated pupils, abdominal cramps, arthralgia/myalgia, hypertension, tachycardia, and craving.
- Treatment includes:
  - Moderate symptoms: Symptomatic treatment with clonidine (for autonomic signs and symptoms of withdrawal), nonsteroidal anti-inflammatory drugs (NSAIDs) for pain, loperamide for diarrhea, dicyclomine for abdominal cramps, etc.
  - Severe symptoms: Detox with buprenorphine or methadone.
  - Monitor degree of withdrawal with COWS (Clinical Opioid Withdrawal Scale), which uses objective measures (i.e., pulse, pupil size, tremor) to assess withdrawal severity.

Hallucinogens

Hallucinogenic drugs of abuse include psilocybin (mushrooms), mescaline (peyote cactus), and lysergic acid diethylamide (LSD). Pharmacological effects vary, but LSD is believed to act on the serotonergic system. Hallucinogens do not cause physical dependence or withdrawal, though users can rarely develop psychological dependence.

INTOXICATION

- Effects include perceptual changes (illusions, hallucinations, body image distortions, synesthesia), labile affect, dilated pupils, tachycardia, hypertension, hyperthermia, tremors, incoordination, sweating, and palpitations.
- Usually lasts 6–12 hours, but may last for several days.
- May have a "bad trip" that consists of marked anxiety, panic, and psychotic symptoms (paranoia, hallucinations).
- **Treatment**: Monitor for dangerous behavior and reassure patient. Use benzodiazepines as first-line for agitation (can use antipsychotics if needed).

WITHDRAWAL

No withdrawal syndrome is produced, but with long-term LSD use, patients may experience flashbacks later in life.

Marijuana

- Cannabis ("marijuana," "pot," "weed," "grass") is the most commonly used illicit substance in the world.
- The main psychoactive component which produces the "high" in cannabis is THC (tetrahydrocannabinol).
- Cannabinoid receptors in the brain inhibit adenylate cyclase.
- Marijuana has shown some efficacy in treating nausea and vomiting in chemotherapy patients, increasing appetite in AIDS patients, in chronic pain (from cancer), and lowering intraocular pressure in glaucoma. A specific class of compounds found in marijuana, cannabidiols (CBDs), is currently being studied for management of pain, seizures, and anxiety/depression.

INTOXICATION

- Marijuana causes euphoria, anxiety, impaired motor coordination, perceptual disturbances (sensation of slowed time), mild tachycardia, anxiety,

conjunctival injection (red eyes), dry mouth, and increased appetite ("the munchies").
- Cannabis-induced psychotic disorders with paranoia, hallucinations, and/or delusions may occur. There is no overdose syndrome for marijuana use.
- Cannabis use disorder occurs in approximately 10% of those who use (up to 50% of daily users).
- Chronic use may cause respiratory problems such as asthma and chronic bronchitis, immunosuppression, cancer, and possible effects on reproductive hormones.
- **Treatment**: Supportive, psychosocial interventions (e.g., contingency management, groups).

WITHDRAWAL

- Withdrawal symptoms may include irritability, anxiety, restlessness, aggression, strange dreams, depression, headaches, sweating, chills, insomnia, and low appetite.
- **Treatment**: Supportive and symptomatic.

> **KEY FACT**
>
> Dronabinol is a pill form of THC that is FDA-approved for certain indications.

Inhalants

- Inhalants include a broad range of drugs that are inhaled and absorbed through the lungs.
- Inhalants generally act as CNS depressants.
- Most commonly used by preadolescents or adolescents; rate of use is similar between boys and girls (but rare in adult females).
- *Examples:* Solvents, glue, paint thinners, fuels, isobutyl nitrates ("huffing," "laughing gas," "rush," "bolt").

INTOXICATION

- **Effects**: Perceptual disturbances, paranoia, lethargy, dizziness, nausea/vomiting, headache, nystagmus, tremor, muscle weakness, hyporeflexia, ataxia, slurred speech, euphoria, hypoxia, clouding of consciousness, stupor, or coma.
- Acute intoxication: 15–30 minutes. May be sustained with repeated use.
- **Overdose**: May be fatal secondary to respiratory depression or cardiac arrhythmias.
- Long-term use may cause permanent damage to CNS (e.g., neurocognitive impairment, cerebellar dysfunction, Parkinsonism, seizures), peripheral neuropathy, myopathy, aplastic anemia, malignancy, metabolic acidosis, urinary calculi, glomerulonephritis, myocarditis, myocardial infarction, and hepatotoxicity.
- **Treatment**: Monitor airway, breathing, and circulation; may need oxygen with hypoxic states.
- Identify solvent because some (e.g., leaded gasoline) may require chelation.

WITHDRAWAL

A withdrawal syndrome does not usually occur, but symptoms may include irritability, sleep disturbance, anxiety, depression, nausea, vomiting, and craving.

Caffeine

Caffeine is the most commonly used psychoactive substance in the United States, usually in the form of coffee, tea, or energy drinks. It acts as an adenosine antagonist, causing increase in cyclic adenosine monophosphate (cAMP) and stimulating the release of excitatory neurotransmitters.

OVERDOSE

- More than 250 mg (2 cups of coffee): Anxiety, insomnia, muscle twitching, rambling speech, flushed face, diuresis, gastrointestinal disturbance, restlessness, excitement, and tachycardia.
- More than 1 g: May cause tinnitus, severe agitation, visual light flashes, and cardiac arrhythmias.
- More than 10 g: Death may occur secondary to seizures and respiratory failure.
- **Treatment**: Supportive and symptomatic.

WITHDRAWAL

- Caffeine withdrawal symptoms occur in 50–75% of caffeine users if cessation is abrupt.
- Withdrawal symptoms include **headache**, fatigue, irritability, nausea, vomiting, drowsiness, muscle pain, and depression.
- Usually resolves within 1½ weeks.

Nicotine

- Nicotine is derived from the tobacco plant, and stimulates nicotinic receptors in autonomic ganglia of the sympathetic and parasympathetic nervous systems. It is highly addictive through its effects on the dopaminergic system.
- Nicotine use causes both tolerance and physical dependence (i.e., prominent craving and withdrawal).
- Cigarette smoking is the leading cause of preventable morbidity and mortality in the United States, posing many health risks including chronic obstructive pulmonary disease (COPD), cardiovascular diseases, and various cancers.
- Current smoking prevalence is about 15% of U.S. adults.
- Effects: Restlessness, insomnia, anxiety, and increase in gastrointestinal motility.
- **Withdrawal symptoms**: Intense craving, dysphoria, anxiety, poor concentration, increase in appetite, weight gain, irritability, restlessness, and insomnia.

WARDS TIP

Cigarette smoking during pregnancy is associated with low birth weight, SIDS, and a variety of postnatal morbidities.

TREATMENT OF NICOTINE DEPENDENCE

FDA-approved pharmacotherapy:

- Varenicline (Chantix): α4β2 nicotinic cholinergic receptor (nAChR) partial agonist that mimics the action of nicotine, reducing the rewarding aspects and preventing withdrawal symptoms.
- Bupropion (Zyban): Antidepressant inhibits reuptake of dopamine and norepinephrine; helps reduce craving and withdrawal symptoms.

- Nicotine replacement therapy (NRT): Available as transdermal patch, gum, lozenge, nasal spray, and inhaler.
- Behavioral support/counseling should be part of every treatment.
- Relapse after abstinence is common.

Gambling Disorder

DIAGNOSIS AND DSM-5 CRITERIA

Persistent and recurrent problematic gambling behavior, as evidenced by four or more of the following in a 12-month period:

1. Preoccupation with gambling.
2. Need to gamble with increasing amount of money to achieve pleasure.
3. Repeated and unsuccessful attempts to cut down on or stop gambling.
4. Restlessness or irritability when attempting to stop gambling.
5. Gambling when feeling distressed (depressed, anxious, etc.).
6. Returning to reclaim losses after gambling ("get even").
7. Lying to hide level of gambling.
8. Jeopardizing relationships or job because of gambling.
9. Relying on others to financially support gambling.

EPIDEMIOLOGY/ETIOLOGY

- Prevalence: 0.4–1.0% of adults in the United States.
- Men represent most of the cases.
- More common in young adults and middle-aged, and lower rates in older adults.
- Similar to substance use disorders, the course is marked by periods of abstinence and relapse.
- Increased incidence of mood disorders, anxiety disorders, substance use disorders, and personality disorders.
- Etiology may involve genetic, temperamental, environmental, and neurochemical factors.
- One-third may achieve recovery without treatment.

TREATMENT

- Participation in Gamblers Anonymous (a 12-step program) is the most common treatment.
- Cognitive behavioral therapy has been shown to be effective, particularly when combined with Gamblers Anonymous.
- Important to treat comorbid mood disorders, anxiety disorders, and substance use disorders where appropriate.

CHAPTER 8

NEUROCOGNITIVE DISORDERS

Definition	98
Delirium	98
Epidemiology	98
Risk Factors	98
Precipitating Factors	98
Etiology	98
Clinical Manifestations	99
Diagnosis	100
Treatment	100
Mild and Major Neurocognitive Disorders	101
Diagnosis	102
Alzheimer Disease (AD)	103
Vascular Disease (Vascular Cognitive Impairment)	104
Lewy Body Disease (LBD)	105
Frontotemporal Degeneration (FTD)	106
HIV Infection	107
Huntington Disease (HD)	107
Parkinson Disease (PD)	108
Prion Disease	109
Normal Pressure Hydrocephalus (NPH)	109

Definition

The neurocognitive disorders (NCDs) comprise a group of conditions defined by a decline from a previous level of cognitive functioning. The six cognitive domains that may be affected include **complex attention**, **executive function**, **learning and memory**, **language**, **perceptual-motor skills**, and **social cognition (interaction)**. By definition, cause(s) for the deficits may be ascertained from findings on history, physical exam, and diagnostic testing. The DSM-5 divides the NCDs into three main categories: delirium, mild NCDs, and major NCDs (dementias).

Delirium

- Delirium is a **medical emergency**.
- May be the only early manifestation of serious illness.
- Potentially reversible. Can advance to coma, seizures, or death.
- Associated with **high mortality**. Up to 40% of individuals die within 1 year of diagnosis.

EPIDEMIOLOGY

- Up to one-half of hospitalized elderly patients develop delirium.
- As many as 90% of patients with a preexisting NCD (dementia) will experience a superimposed delirium when admitted to the hospital.
- Delirium often goes unrecognized (65–88% of the time).

RISK FACTORS

- Advanced age.
- Preexisting cognitive impairment or depression.
- Prior history of delirium.
- Severe or terminal illness.
- Multiple medical comorbidities.
- Hearing or vision impairment.

PRECIPITATING FACTORS

- Polypharmacy, including the use of psychotropic medications (especially benzodiazepines and anticholinergic drugs).
- Alcohol use or withdrawal.
- Infection.
- Pain.
- Dehydration.
- Malnutrition.
- Impaired mobility.
- Sleep deprivation.
- Organ failure.

ETIOLOGY

- Almost any medical condition can cause delirium (see examples in Table 8-1).
- The DSM-5 recognizes five broad categories:
  - Substance intoxication delirium.

WARDS TIP

Terms commonly used for delirium include *toxic or metabolic encephalopathy*, *acute organic brain syndrome*, *acute confusional state*, *acute toxic psychosis*, and *ICU psychosis*.

WARDS TIP

Consider delirium as acute brain failure—a *medical emergency* like other acute organ failures.

WARDS TIP

The "ICU triad" includes delirium, pain, and agitation. All three of these interdependent conditions must be addressed.

WARDS TIP

Delirium is commonly experienced by patients in the ICU and postoperative recovery.

TABLE 8-1. Clinical Scenarios of Delirium on Exam

Scenario	Likely Diagnosis	Diagnostic Testing
Delirium + fever + cough + rales	Pneumonia	Chest x-ray
Delirium + dysuria + suprapubic tenderness	Urinary tract infection	Urinalysis and urine culture
Delirium + constricted pupils (miosis) + bradypnea	Opioid intoxication	Urine toxicology screen
Delirium + fever + nuchal rigidity + photophobia	Meningitis	Lumbar puncture
Delirium + tachycardia + tremor + thyromegaly	Thyrotoxicosis	TSH, free T_4, T_3
Delirium + insulin use	Hypoglycemia	Blood glucose

- Substance withdrawal delirium.
- Medication-induced delirium.
- Delirium due to another medical condition.
- Delirium due to multiple etiologies.

CLINICAL MANIFESTATIONS

- Primarily a disorder of **attention** and **awareness** (i.e., **orientation**).
- Cognitive deficits **develop acutely** over hours to days.
- Symptoms **fluctuate** throughout the course of a day, typically worsening at night.
- Other features include deficits in **recent memory**, language abnormalities, or perceptual disturbances (usually **visual**, such as illusions or hallucinations).
- Circadian rhythm disruption and emotional symptoms are common.
- There are three types of delirium based on psychomotor activity.
  - Mixed type
    - Psychomotor activity may remain stable at baseline or fluctuate rapidly between hyperactivity and hypoactivity.
    - **Most common** type.
  - Hypoactive ("quiet") type
    - Decreased psychomotor activity, ranging from drowsiness to lethargy to stupor.
    - **More likely to go undetected.**
    - More common in the elderly.
  - Hyperactive type ("ICU psychosis")
    - Manifests with agitation, mood lability, and uncooperativeness.
    - Less common, but more easily identified due to its disruptiveness.
    - More common in **drug withdrawal or toxicity**.
- Hospitalized patients usually recover within 1 week, although some degree of cognitive deficits can persist for months or even indefinitely.

WARDS TIP

Common causes of medication-induced delirium:
- Tricyclic antidepressants
- Anticholinergics
- Benzodiazepines
- Nonbenzodiazepine hypnotics ("Z-drugs")
- Corticosteroids
- H2 blockers
- Opioids (especially meperidine)

WARDS TIP

The most common precipitants of delirium in children are febrile illnesses and medications.

WARDS TIP

Suspect delirium if a patient presents with altered mental status, disorientation, confusion, agitation, or sudden-onset of psychotic symptoms.

WARDS TIP

A quick, first-glance bedside exam for suspected substance/medication intoxication is **VALEUMS**.
- **V**ital signs
- **A**lertness **L**evel
- **E**yes (pupil size and position)
- **U**rine (bladder distention or incontinence)
- **M**ucous membranes (moisture)
- **S**kin (temperature and moisture)

KEY FACT

Delirium generally manifests as diffuse background slowing on electroencephalography (EEG). An exception to this is the case of delirium tremens, which is associated with fast EEG activity. EEG lacks sensitivity and specificity for making the diagnosis, but is useful for ruling out nonconvulsive seizures.

WARDS TIP

Consider obtaining a head CT for a patient with delirium under the following circumstances:
- No underlying cause evident on initial evaluation.
- In the context of head trauma.
- New focal neurologic deficits detected on exam.
- Patient unable or unwilling to cooperate with a neurologic examination.
- No improvement despite treatment of already identified causes.

TABLE 8-2. DSM-5 Criteria for Delirium

- Disturbance in **attention** and **awareness**.
- Disturbance in **an additional cognitive domain**.
- Develops **acutely** over hours to days, represents a **change** from baseline, and tends to **fluctuate**.
- **Not** better accounted for by **another neurocognitive disorder**.
- **Not** occurring during a **coma**.
- Evidence from history, physical, or labs that the disturbance is a **direct consequence** of **another medical condition**, **substance intoxication/withdrawal**, exposure to **toxin**, or due to multiple etiologies.

DIAGNOSIS

- Table 8-2 summarizes the DSM-5 diagnostic criteria.
- A useful clinical tool for evaluation of a patient with suspected delirium is the **Confusion Assessment Method** (CAM).
    - This method takes only 5 minutes to perform and has a high sensitivity and specificity.
    - Delirium is diagnosed in a patient with **inattention** of **acute onset** and/or **fluctuating course** along with either **disorganized thinking** or **altered consciousness**.
        - Inattention manifests as distractibility or difficulty maintaining focus during the evaluation.
        - Disorganized thinking is demonstrated via derailment or loose associations.
        - Level of consciousness ranges from vigilant (hyperalert) to alert (normal) to lethargic (drowsy, but easily aroused) to stuporous (difficult to arouse) to comatose (unarousable to verbal stimulation).
- Once delirium has been diagnosed, the cause(s) should be sought.
    - Finger-stick blood glucose, pulse-oximetry, arterial blood gases, and electrocardiography can quickly provide useful data at bedside.
    - Labs typically obtained in a delirium workup include a basic metabolic panel, complete blood count with differential, urinalysis, and urine culture.
    - Urine drug screen, a blood alcohol level, therapeutic drug levels (e.g., antiepileptics, digoxin, lithium), a hepatic panel, thyroid hormone levels, or a chest x-ray may also be warranted depending on the clinical presentation.
    - Head imaging (head CT or MRI brain), EEG, and lumbar puncture should be performed if focal neurological deficits are present or a cause of delirium cannot be identified with the initial workup.

TREATMENT

- **Treat the underlying cause(s)**.
- Address potential exacerbating factors: Mobility limitations, sensory deficits, sleep cycle disruption, constipation, urinary retention, dehydration, electrolyte abnormalities, uncontrolled pain, and medications.

- Encourage a family member to stay at the bedside to help with supervision.
- Utilize a one-to-one sitter if needed.
- Reorient the patient on a regular basis regarding time, place, and situation. For example, open window blinds during the day and place whiteboards, calendars, and clocks in plain sight.
- D2 antagonists (i.e., antipsychotics) are indicated for treatment of agitation that endangers the patient or others.
- **Haloperidol** is the preferred agent and can be administered orally, intramuscularly, or intravenously.
- D2 antagonists exacerbate extrapyramidal symptoms; use with caution in patients with Parkinsonism.
- Avoid the use of restraints. They can worsen agitation and cause injury. When restraints are necessary, reassess often and remove as soon as possible. Use the least restrictive means appropriate for the situation.

An 83-year-old woman is admitted to the hospital after presenting with a fever and altered mental status. Her home nurse aide reports that the patient was in her usual state of health until 24 hours prior to admission when she became confused and seemed to be talking to herself. In a few hours, her mental status improved then deteriorated again. After the patient dialed 911 to report that she was being held hostage by terrorists, her nurse aid called an ambulance on her behalf.

On examination, the patient is somnolent and has difficulty responding to questions appropriately. She is disoriented to place and time.

When the daughter calls to check in, she shares that her mother has had progressive memory deficits over the past several years. The patient can no longer drive and requires assistance with finances and meal preparation.

What is the most likely diagnosis?

The patient most likely has delirium. She presents with a sudden change in cognition as manifested by confusion, disorientation, and hallucinations. She has had an acute change from her baseline behavior. Her symptoms wax and wane throughout the day, representing the typical fluctuation found in delirium. She presents with a fever, likely secondary to an infection which caused her symptoms. If confirmed, her diagnosis would be delirium due to the specific infectious etiology.

Collateral information points to a prior diagnosis of major neurocognitive disorder (dementia). She has a history of memory impairment that began gradually and has progressively worsened. There is also history of impairment in executive functioning, and she can no longer care for herself. The existence of a major neurocognitive disorder is a risk factor for the development of a superimposed delirium.

WARDS TIP

Generally avoid using benzodiazepines to treat delirium. These medications often worsen delirium by causing paradoxical disinhibition or oversedation. Prescribe only in the case of delirium due to alcohol or benzodiazepine withdrawal.

Mild and Major Neurocognitive Disorders

- The non-delirium NCDs are characterized by a chronic cognitive decline that impacts functioning in daily activities (Table 8-3).

TABLE 8-3. DSM-5 Criteria for Mild and Major NCDs

Criterion	Mild NCDs	Major NCDs
Functional decline in at least one cognitive domain relative to baseline as evidenced by		
Concern (expressed by the patient or someone who knows them)	Mild decline	Significant decline
Objective findings on cognitive testing (preferably standardized neuropsychological testing)	Modest impairment	Substantial impairment
Effect on functioning in daily life.	Ability to perform IADLs preserved	Impaired performance of IADLs/ADLs
Deficits do not occur exclusively in the context of a delirium		
Deficits are not better explained by another mental disorder.		

ADLs, basic activities of daily living; IADLs, independent activities of daily living.

- Individuals with **mild NCDs** (aka mild cognitive impairment) experience difficulty with some of the more complex activities of daily living but are able to maintain their independence.
- Patients with **major NCDs** require assistance with independent activities of daily living (IADLs), such as paying bills, managing medications, or shopping for groceries. Over time, the basic activities of daily living (e.g., feeding, toileting, bathing) are affected, eventually leading to total dependence.
- The mild and major NCDs are also subcategorized by etiology (Table 8-4).
  - The **dementias** comprise a large group of progressive and irreversible major NCDs that primarily affect the elderly.
  - Several other major NCDs present similarly to the dementias, but their progression may be arrested or even reversed with treatment (e.g., vitamin B_{12} deficiency, thyroid dysfunction, normal pressure hydrocephalus).

KEY FACT

Thyroid dysfunction can cause reversible cognitive impairment. Hypothyroidism is typically accompanied by fatigue and cold intolerance. Hyperthyroidism in the elderly may manifest as an "apathetic thyrotoxicosis," characterized by depression and lethargy. Thyroid function tests are typically included in the initial evaluation of any psychiatric illness.

DIAGNOSIS

- The **Mini Mental State Exam (MMSE)** is a screening test used due to its speed and ease of administration.
  - Assesses orientation, attention/concentration, language, constructional ability, and immediate and delayed recall.
  - Sensitive for major NCDs (e.g., dementias), particularly moderate-to-severe forms.
    - Perfect score: 30.
    - Dysfunction: <25.
  - Not as sensitive for mild NCDs and early major NCDs.
  - Lacks specificity.
  - Norm tables are available to adjust for age and education.
- Another commonly used screening tool is the **Mini-Cog**.
  - Consists of three-item recall and clock-drawing tasks.
  - Positive screening for cognitive impairment:
    - No items recalled after 3 minutes.

TABLE 8-4. Clinical Scenarios of Mild or Major Neurocognitive Disorder on Exam

Scenario	Likely Diagnosis	Diagnostic Testing
Cognitive impairment with stepwise increase in severity + focal neurological signs	Vascular disease	Head CT/Brain MRI
Cognitive impairment + cogwheel rigidity + resting tremor	Lewy body disease Parkinson disease	Clinical exam
Cognitive impairment + gait apraxia + urinary incontinence	Normal pressure hydrocephalus	Head CT/Brain MRI
Cognitive impairment + fatigue + cold intolerance	Hypothyroidism	TSH, free T_4
Cognitive impairment + vegan diet + paresthesias + diminished position and vibration sensation	Vitamin B_{12} deficiency	Serum B_{12}
Cognitive impairment + tremor + Kayser–Fleischer rings	Wilson disease	Ceruloplasmin
Cognitive impairment + diminished position and vibration sensation + **A**rgyll **R**obertson **P**upils (**A**ccommodation **R**esponse **P**resent, response to light absent)	Neurosyphilis	CSF FTA-ABS and VDRL

CSF, cerebrospinal fluid; CT, computed tomography; FTA-ABS, fluorescent treponemal antibody absorption test; MRI, magnetic resonance imaging; T_4, thyroxine; TSH, thyroid-stimulating hormone; VDRL, Venereal Disease Research Laboratory.

- Only one to two items recalled with abnormal clock drawing.
- Negative screening:
  - All three items repeated correctly after 3 minutes.
  - One to two items recalled with normal clock drawing.
- Other commonly used screening tools include:
  - Blessed Orientation-Memory-Concentration (BOMC).
  - Montreal Cognitive Assessment (MoCA).
  - Frontal Assessment Battery (FAB).
- An abnormal screening test indicates the need for further testing, preferably formal neuropsychological testing.

ALZHEIMER DISEASE (AD)

Alzheimer disease is the **most common** underlying etiology of major NCDs (dementias).

Clinical Manifestations

- **Gradual progressive decline** in cognitive functions.
- The primary cognitive domains affected are **memory**, **learning**, and **language**.
- Personality changes, mood swings, and paranoia are very common.
- Motor and sensory symptoms appear in advanced disease.
- On average, death occurs 10 years after diagnosis.

KEY FACT

Postmortem pathological examination of the brain is the only way to definitively diagnose Alzheimer disease.

KEY FACT

Senile plaques and neurofibrillary tangles are not only found in Alzheimer disease, but also in Down syndrome and even in normal aging.

KEY FACT

Adults with Down syndrome are at increased risk of developing Alzheimer disease in midlife.

WARDS TIP

Antipsychotics carry a black box warning about increased risk of death in patients with dementia.

Diagnosis

- A diagnosis of **possible** NCD due to AD is made based on the presence of characteristic clinical findings:
    - Insidious onset.
    - Gradual progression.
    - Impairment in one (mild NCD) or more (major NCD) cognitive domains.
- NCD due to AD is **probable** if there is evidence of causation by one of several single-gene variants.

Etiology

- Accumulation of extraneuronal *beta*-amyloid plaques and intraneuronal *tau* protein tangles is associated with progressive brain atrophy.
- Approximately 1% of AD results from an autosomal dominant single-gene mutation (amyloid precursor protein, presenilin 1, or presenilin 2), which is associated with an early onset of symptoms.
- The *epsilon*-4 variant of the *apolipoprotein* gene is a risk factor for developing early-onset AD.

Epidemiology

- AD pathology is estimated to play a role in 60–90% of major NCDs.
- Approximately 50% of patients with AD pathology actually have an NCD due to multiple etiologies.
- Two-thirds of patients diagnosed with AD are women.
- Diagnosed after the age of 65 in the vast majority of individuals.

Treatment

- No cure or truly effective treatment.
- **Cholinesterase inhibitors** (e.g., donepezil, rivastigmine, and galantamine) may slow clinical deterioration by 6–12 months in up to 50% of patients with mild-to-moderate AD.
- The **NMDA receptor antagonist**, memantine, may provide a modest benefit to patients with moderate-to-severe disease.
- Antipsychotic medications are often used to treat agitation and aggression.
    - Because they are associated with **increased mortality** in patients with dementia, low doses should be prescribed for short periods of time.
    - Ideally, informed consent should be obtained from patients and/or their designated decision makers.
    - **Monitor closely** for side effects.
- Supportive care via behavioral, social, and environmental interventions.
- A **multidisciplinary approach** is necessary.
- Any treatment plan must include **caregiver support**.

VASCULAR DISEASE (VASCULAR COGNITIVE IMPAIRMENT)

- Second most common single cause of major NCD after AD, accounting for approximately 20% of major NCDs.
- Evidence of vascular disease is found in $1/2$ of all major NCDs, most commonly comorbid with AD pathology (NCD due to multiple etiologies).
- Cognitive decline occurs as a result of at least one of the following mechanisms:
    - Large vessel strokes, usually cortical.
    - Small vessel strokes (lacunar infarcts) to subcortical structures.
    - Microvascular disease affecting the periventricular white matter.
- Effects vary based on the size, location, and number of infarcts.

Risk Factors
- Hypertension.
- Diabetes.
- Smoking.
- Obesity.
- Hyperlipidemia.
- Atrial fibrillation.
- Advanced age.

Clinical Manifestations
- Presentation and progression of cognitive impairment are variable.
  - Classically demonstrates a stepwise deterioration corresponding with the occurrence of micro-infarcts (i.e., multi-infarct dementia).
  - May present with acute onset followed by partial improvement.
  - May have an insidious onset with gradual decline similar to AD.
- **Complex attention** and **executive functions** are the cognitive domains typically affected in small vessel disease.
- Confirmation of the diagnosis requires neuroimaging with findings that correlate to the clinical picture.

Treatment
- No cure or truly effective treatment.
- Manage risk factors with a goal of preventing future strokes.
- Symptomatic treatment is similar to AD.

> **KEY FACT**
>
> A lesion to the frontal lobe can manifest with a spectrum of symptoms including personality changes, disinhibition, inappropriate behavior, aggression, apathy, amotivation, and paranoia.

> A 68-year-old woman is brought to the clinic by her husband. He reports that his wife has recently seemed confused and has been overly emotional. The patient is able to complete her daily activities at home, but reports some increased difficulty with planning and decision-making. Her medical history is significant for hypertension and transient ischemic attacks (TIAs). A physical exam reveals a carotid bruit.
>
> ***What is the likely diagnosis?*** **Mild vascular NCD.**

LEWY BODY DISEASE (LBD)

As reflected in its name, the major pathologic features of LBD are Lewy bodies (pathologic aggregations of *alpha*-synuclein) and Lewy neurites in the brain, primarily in the basal ganglia.

Clinical Manifestations
- Progressive cognitive decline.
- Commonly coexists with AD and/or cerebrovascular disease as NCD due to multiple etiologies.
- Core features:
  - **Waxing and waning** of cognition, especially in the areas of **attention** and **alertness**.
  - **Visual hallucinations**—usually vivid, colorful, well-formed images of animals or small people.
  - **Rapid eye movement** (REM) **sleep behavior disorder** (not currently included in the DSM-5 core features)—violent movements during sleep in response to dreams, often of fighting.

- Development of **extrapyramidal signs** (Parkinsonism) at least 1 year after cognitive decline becomes evident.
- Suggestive features:
  - Pronounced **antipsychotic sensitivity** (i.e., extra-pyramidal symptoms).
  - Postural instability and recurrent falls.
  - Loss of consciousness or transient unresponsiveness.
  - Autonomic dysfunction.
  - Diminished sense of smell.
  - Non-visual hallucinations and delusions.
  - Excessive sleepiness.
  - Depression, anxiety, and apathy.
- Indicative biomarkers:
  - REM sleep without atonia (RWSA) demonstrated via polysomnography.
  - Decreased 123iodine-MIBG uptake on myocardial scintigraphy.
  - Evidence of reduced dopamine receptor uptake in the basal ganglia via SPECT or PET.

Diagnosis

- Definitive diagnosis can only be made with autopsy.
- **Possible** NCD with Lewy bodies: Only one core feature without evidence from indicative biomarkers OR one or more indicative biomarker(s), but no core clinical features.
- **Probable** NCD with Lewy bodies: Two or more core features OR one core feature and one or more indicative biomarker(s).

Treatment

- **Cholinesterase inhibitors** for cognitive and behavioral symptoms.
- **Quetiapine** or **clozapine** for psychotic symptoms.
  - Use the lowest effective dose for the shortest period of time possible.
  - Monitor closely for adverse effects, such as extrapyramidal signs, sedation, increased confusion, autonomic dysfunction, and signs of **Neuroleptic Malignant Syndrome (NMS)**.
- Levodopa-carbidopa for Parkinsonism.
  - Not as effective as in idiopathic Parkinson disease.
  - May exacerbate psychosis or REM sleep behavior disorder.
- Melatonin and/or clonazepam for REM sleep behavior disorder.

FRONTOTEMPORAL DEGENERATION (FTD)

- FTD includes a diverse group of clinical and pathological disorders that typically present between the ages of 45 and 65.
- Approximately 40% are familial, and 10% are autosomal dominant.

Clinical Manifestations

- Cognitive deficits in **attention**, **abstraction**, **planning**, and **problem solving**.
- **Behavioral variant:**
  - **Disinhibited** verbal, physical, or sexual behavior.
  - Overeating or oral exploration of inanimate objects.
  - Lack of emotional warmth, empathy, or sympathy.
  - Apathy or inertia.
  - Perseveration, repetitive speech, rituals, or obsessions.
  - Decline in **social cognition** and/or **executive abilities**.
- **Language variant** (primary progressive aphasia):
  - Difficulties with **speech** and **comprehension**.

- Relative sparing of learning/memory and perceptual-motor function.
- Many individuals have features of both the behavioral and language variants.
- Increased sensitivity to adverse effects of antipsychotics.

Pathology
Marked atrophy of the frontal and temporal lobes.

Diagnosis
- Definitive diagnosis cannot be made until autopsy.
- FTD is **probable** if frontotemporal atrophy is evident on structural imaging or hypoactivity is visualized on functional imaging in context of the characteristic clinical signs.

Treatment
- Symptom-focused.
- Serotonergic medications (e.g., SSRIs, trazodone) may help reduce disinhibition, anxiety, impulsivity, repetitive behaviors, and eating disorders.

HIV INFECTION

- HIV is the most common infectious agent known to cause cognitive impairment.
- In HIV+ patients, 33% have asymptomatic neurocognitive impairment that appears on exam, 12% have mild NCD, and 2% have major NCD.
- Severe forms of NCD due to HIV infection have become much less common with the widespread use of antiretroviral drugs.

Risk Factors
- History of severe immunosuppression.
- High viral loads in the CSF.
- Advanced HIV infection.

Clinical Manifestations
- Variable presentation depending on the part(s) of the brain affected.
- Decline may be observed in executive functioning, attention, working memory, and psychomotor activity.
- Psychiatric and neuromotor symptoms may also be present.

Diagnosis
Mild or major NCD attributable to confirmed HIV infection.

Treatment
- Antiretroviral therapy (ART) improves cognition in some patients.
- Psychostimulants target fatigue, apathy, and psychomotor retardation.

HUNTINGTON DISEASE (HD)

- A genetic disorder resulting from trinucleotide (CAG) repeats in the gene encoding the huntingtin (HTT) protein on chromosome 4.
- Autosomal dominant mode of inheritance.

Clinical Manifestations

- Characterized by a triad of **motor**, **cognitive**, and **psychiatric** symptoms.
- Average age at diagnosis is 40 years.
- Cognitive decline and behavioral changes can precede onset of motor signs by up to 15 years.
- **Executive function** is the primary cognitive domain affected.
- Psychiatric manifestations include depression, apathy, irritability, obsessions, impulsivity, paranoia, delusions, and hallucinations.
- Patients are often aware of deteriorating mentation.
- Increased rate of suicide (7%).
- Movement disorders include **chorea** (jerky, dance-like movements) and **bradykinesia**.

Diagnosis

- Extrapyramidal movement disorder in an individual with either a **family history** of HD or **genetic testing** that confirms an increased number of CAG repeats in the HTT gene.
- Mild or major NCD may be diagnosed prior to onset of motor signs if an individual is determined to be at risk based on family history or genetic testing.

Treatment

Symptom-directed therapy with **tetrabenazine** or **atypical (second-generation) antipsychotics**.

PARKINSON DISEASE (PD)

- An idiopathic, progressive neurodegenerative disease characterized by depletion of dopamine in the basal ganglia.
- Up to 75% of patients with PD meet the criteria for major NCD, typically in advanced disease.

Clinical Manifestations

- Motor signs include rigidity, resting tremor, bradykinesia, and postural instability.
- Cognitive manifestations consist of executive dysfunction and visuospatial impairments.
- Depression, anxiety, personality changes, and apathy are common.
- Psychotic symptoms, including visual hallucinations and paranoid delusions, may result from the disease itself or from adverse effects of the medications used to treat the motor symptoms.

Diagnosis

- Diagnosis of PD requires the presence of **bradykinesia** and either **tremor** or **rigidity**.
- Associated with asymmetry of motor symptoms and favorable response to dopaminergic therapy.
- Mild or major NCD is attributed to PD if **cognitive decline appears after the onset of motor symptoms** and no other underlying etiology is identified.

Treatment

- Motor symptoms are most commonly treated with **carbidopa-levodopa** and/or **dopamine agonists**.

- Cholinesterase inhibitors are used to target cognitive symptoms and may also ameliorate some of the neuropsychiatric symptoms (hallucinations).
- Psychotic symptoms may respond to a reduction in the dose of dopamine agonists.
- **Low dose quetiapine** and **clozapine** are the preferred medications for treatment of psychotic symptoms. Avoid other antipsychotics since they can worsen the motor symptoms of PD.

> **KEY FACT**
>
> Symptoms of Parkinson disease can be exacerbated by antipsychotic medications.

PRION DISEASE

- A form of subacute spongiform encephalopathy caused by *pro*teinaceous *in*fectious particles (prions).
- Most cases occur sporadically.
- The most common type is **Creutzfeldt–Jakob disease**.
- Up to 15% are familial (autosomal dominant).
- Less than 1% are iatrogenic.

Clinical Manifestations

- Insidious onset with **rapidly progressive** cognitive decline.
- Difficulties with **concentration**, **memory**, and **judgment** occur early.
- More than 90% of patients experience **myoclonus** (often provoked by startle) at some point in the illness.
- Depression, apathy, and hypersomnia are also common.
- Basal ganglia and cerebellar dysfunction, manifesting as **ataxia**, **nystagmus**, and **hypokinesia**, are present in a majority of individuals.

> **KEY FACT**
>
> Rapidly progressive cognitive decline with myoclonus is suggestive of Creutzfeldt–Jakob disease.

Diagnosis

- Definitive diagnosis requires analysis of brain tissue obtained via biopsy or autopsy.
- A diagnosis of probable CJD requires:
  - **Rapid progression** of cognitive decline.
  - At least two of the following typical clinical features.
    - **Myoclonus.**
    - Visual or cerebellar signs.
    - Pyramidal or extrapyramidal signs.
    - Akinetic mutism.
  - Supportive findings from at least one diagnostic modality.
    - Periodic sharp wave complexes on EEG.
    - CSF positive for 14-3-3 proteins.
    - Lesions in the putamen or caudate nucleus on MRI.

Treatment

- No effective treatment exists.
- Most individuals die within 1 year of diagnosis.

NORMAL PRESSURE HYDROCEPHALUS (NPH)

- NPH is a potentially reversible cause of cognitive dysfunction.
- Enlarged ventricles (on imaging) with a **localized elevation** of cerebrospinal fluid (CSF) pressure but **normal opening pressures** on lumbar puncture.
- The etiology is either idiopathic or secondary to obstruction of CSF reabsorption sites due to infection (meningitis) or hemorrhage (subarachnoid or intraventricular).

KEY FACT

The 3 Ws of NPH
Wobbly = Gait disturbance
Wet = Urinary incontinence
Wacky = Cognitive impairment

Clinical Manifestations

- Classically presents with a clinical triad:
    - **Gait disturbance** ("Wobbly").
        - Most likely to be the first manifestation.
        - Slow with short steps.
        - Broad-based with outwardly rotated feet.
        - Feet appear to be stuck to the floor.
        - Postural instability leads to recurrent falls.
    - **Urinary incontinence** ("Wet").
        - May begin as urinary urgency.
        - Gait disturbance may interfere with reaching the toilet before loss of urine.
        - In later stages, apathy may contribute.
    - **Cognitive impairment** ("Wacky").
        - Insidious onset.
        - Executive dysfunction.
        - Psychomotor retardation.
        - Decreased attention.
        - Apathy.
- Neuroimaging shows enlargement of ventricles out of proportion to cortical atrophy.
- Clinical improvement with CSF removal via lumbar puncture.

Treatment

- Placement of a shunt (usually ventriculoperitoneal) may improve symptoms.
- Cognitive impairment is least likely to improve.

CHAPTER 9

GERIATRIC PSYCHIATRY

Normal Aging	112
Major Depression	112
Pseudodementia	112
Treatment	112
Bereavement	115
Substance Use	115
Psychiatric Manifestations of Major Neurocognitive Disorders (Dementia)	116
Treatment	117
Sleep Disturbance	117
Other Issues	118
Restraints	118
Medications	118
Elder Abuse	118
Nursing Homes	118

The geriatric population of the United States is projected to more than double by the year 2050, boosted in a large part by the aging Baby Boomer generation. Nearly 20% of people over the age of 60 have a psychiatric disorder. The suicide rate of elderly (aged 85 and older) white men is five times the national average.

Common diagnoses in elderly patients include mood disorders, anxiety disorders, and neurocognitive disorders, though many mental disorders in this population remain underreported.

Normal Aging

Factors associated with normal aging include:

- Decreased brain weight/enlarged ventricles and sulci.
- Decreased muscle mass/increased fat.
- Impaired vision and hearing.
- Minor forgetfulness (sometimes called age-associated memory impairment or benign senescent forgetfulness).

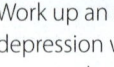

WARDS TIP

Work up an elderly patient for major depression when he/she presents with memory loss or nonspecific physical complaints.

Major Depression

Major depression is a common mental disorder in the geriatric population, with depressive symptoms present in 5–15% of the elderly. Depression is associated with poor physical health:

- Post-myocardial infarction (MI) patients who develop depression have a four times increased rate of death.
- Stroke patients who develop depression have a more than three times increased rate of death during the 10 years following their stroke.
- New admits to nursing homes suffering from depression have increased in 1-year mortality rate.

Pseudodementia

WARDS TIP

Patients with a major neurocognitive disorder are more likely to confabulate when they do not know an answer, whereas depressed patients may just say that they don't know. When pressed for an answer, depressed patients will often show the capacity to answer correctly.

Symptoms of major depression in the elderly often include problems with memory and cognitive functioning. Because this clinical picture may be mistaken for a major neurocognitive disorder (dementia), it is termed *pseudodementia*.

Pseudodementia is the presence of apparent cognitive deficits in patients with major depression. Patients may appear to be suffering from a neurocognitive disorder (dementia). However, their symptoms are secondary to their underlying depression, and it can be difficult to differentiate the two (see Table 9-1).

TREATMENT

- Supportive psychotherapy.
- Community resources: Senior centers, senior services, support groups, etc.
- Antidepressant medications (selective serotonin reuptake inhibitors [SSRIs] and other newer antidepressants have fewer side effects and are

TABLE 9-1. Dementia Versus Pseudodementia (Depression)

Dementia	Pseudodementia (Depression)
Onset is insidious.	Onset is more acute.
Sundowning is common (↑ confusion at night).	Sundowning is uncommon.
Will guess at answers (confabulate).	Often answers "I don't know."
Patient is unaware of problems.	Patient is aware of problems.
Cognitive deficits do not improve with antidepressant treatment.	Cognitive deficits improve with antidepressants.

preferable to tricyclic antidepressants [TCAs] or monoamine oxidase [MAO] inhibitors).
- Elderly patients are sensitive to side effects of medications so it's important to start at a very low dose and titrate slowly up to the full dose of the antidepressant.
- If using TCAs in elderly patients, nortriptyline is favored because it has the fewest anticholinergic side effects.
- Mirtazapine can increase appetite and is also sedating; it is dosed at bedtime for depressed patients who particularly suffer from decreased appetite and sleep disturbances.
- Methylphenidate can be used at low doses as an adjunct to antidepressants for patients with severe depression and/or psychomotor retardation; however, it may cause insomnia if given in the afternoon or evening. Also, be aware of the risk of arrhythmia in patients with cardiac disease.
- Electroconvulsive therapy (ECT) may be used in place of antidepressants (ECT is safe and effective in the elderly).

KEY FACT

The most common psychiatric disorder in the elderly is major depressive disorder.

KEY FACT

White elderly males have the highest rate of completed suicides.

Mrs. Brennan is a 72-year-old Caucasian woman who considers herself to be in good health. She goes out to lunch with friends three times a week and looks forward to her Saturday bridge games at the local senior center. Unfortunately, her husband has suffered from years of ill health, including five myocardial infarctions and a serious stroke last year that left him barely able to walk. You are a geriatric psychiatrist who has been treating Mrs. Brennan's husband for depression that began after his last stroke. Mrs. Brennan always comes along to appointments so that she can stay informed about her husband's medical care.

You become concerned when your patient uncharacteristically misses an appointment and does not return your phone message. Finally, a month later, you are surprised to see Mrs. Brennan walk into your office alone. She enters the room slowly, and you notice that she has lost some weight since you last saw her.

She sits down but does not make eye contact. Finally, she begins to talk in a soft, monotone voice, explaining that her husband had another bad stroke last month and was moved to a hospice facility, where he passed away 2 weeks ago. She begins to cry, and you hand her some tissues.

The two of you talk some more about her husband's death and how she is coping with it. She reports that her daughter visits her frequently and has invited her to spend the weekends with her.

Although Mrs. Brennan reports that she feels "down," she reports that she is making an effort to go on with her life because that is what her husband would have wanted. She says that she went out to lunch with her friends this week and adds that they are very supportive. Mrs. Brennan also reports that it is difficult for her to realize that her husband is no longer there and says that she has heard his voice calling her a couple of times this week. As she leaves your office, you tell her she is welcome to come back whenever she wants.

Is Mrs. Brennan having a normal grief reaction?

Yes, Mrs. Brennan is going through a normal grieving process, also known as bereavement. Although she displays some symptoms suggestive of major depression (psychomotor retardation, depressed mood), and reports the presence of auditory hallucinations (her husband's voice), these symptoms are commonly encountered in bereavement and are considered a normal reaction to her sudden loss.

Three months later, you receive a phone call from Mrs. Brennan's daughter, who expresses concern about her mother. She tells you that her mother has to be urged to shower, wear clean clothes, and eat regularly. Mrs. Brennan has stopped participating in her bridge group and has not been out with her friends in many weeks. The daughter also worries about Mrs. Brennan's increasing forgetfulness and memory problems. She asks if she can bring her in for an appointment with you. You agree immediately and schedule Mrs. Brennan the next day.

Mrs. Brennan enters your office with her daughter by her side. She is dressed in a wrinkled pantsuit and is wearing scuffed shoes. Her hair is clean but lies limply against her head. She appears much thinner than the last time you saw her. Her eyes are downcast, and she appears sad. You try to engage her in conversation, but her answers to your questions are soft and short. When you do an assessment of her memory, you note that she answers basic questions with "I don't know" and scores poorly on the mini-mental state exam questions.

What is Mrs. Brennan's most likely diagnosis now?

Mrs. Brennan is most likely suffering from a major depressive episode. Her symptoms now fulfill criteria for major depressive disorder and have been present for over 2 weeks. Since her memory problems began after she began experiencing depressive symptoms, these are likely secondary to depression. When this occurs, it is often referred to as "pseudodementia." If this is the case, as her depression is treated her memory deficits will improve.

What are possible treatment options for Mrs. Brennan?

Supportive psychotherapy and a medication trial of an SSRI would be excellent first-line treatments. In addition, you suggest to Mrs. Brennan and her daughter to consider visiting her local senior center to learn what kinds of services she might benefit from.

Bereavement

In 1969, Elisabeth Kübler-Ross, MD, published a book called *On Death and Dying*, in which she proposed a model of bereavement, the Five Stages of Grief.

- **Denial:** *"This isn't happening to me. I don't feel sick."*
- **Anger:** *"It's my ex-husband's fault for smoking around me all those years!"*
- **Bargaining:** *"Maybe if I exercise and improve my diet, I'll get better."*
- **Depression:** *"There's no hope for a cure. I will die of this cancer."*
- **Acceptance:** *"I may have cancer, but I've always been a fighter—why stop now?"*

There is some controversy surrounding this model (e.g., people may not experience all of the stages or they may go through them in a different order) as grief is a very individualized experience; there is no "correct" way to mourn a loss. However, it is important to be able to distinguish normal grief reactions from unhealthy, pathological ones.

- **Normal grief** may involve many intense feelings, including guilt and sadness, sleep disturbances, appetite changes, and illusions/hallucinations (not always pathological in some cultures). These feelings generally abate within 6 months of the loss, and the patient's ability to function appropriately in their life is preserved.
- **Bereavement-associated depression** is a major depression that begins with a concrete death or loss in the patient's life. It is often difficult to distinguish between depression and grief, since many symptoms are similar.
    - Look for generalized feelings of hopelessness, helplessness, severe guilt and worthlessness, neurovegetative symptoms (e.g., insomnia, appetite/weight changes, low energy), and suicidal ideation, in addition to grief symptoms.
    - Treatment for depression is recommended in patients who have at least 2 weeks of persistent depressive symptoms.

WARDS TIP

The elderly are very sensitive to side effects of medications, particularly anticholinergic effects of antidepressants.

Substance Use

- Forty percent of the 65 plus-year-old population drink alcohol, and up to 16% are heavy drinkers who may experience adverse health events from the amount of alcohol they use or from its interaction with medications and impact on chronic disease processes. It is important to screen elderly patients for substance use.
- Age-related effects of alcohol:
    - Elderly people have a lower amount of alcohol dehydrogenase in their livers which can lead to higher blood alcohol levels (BALs) with fewer drinks as compared to younger adults.
    - The amount of water in the body lessens with age, resulting in a higher percentage of alcohol in the blood of elderly compared to younger people after drinking the same amount of alcohol.
    - The central nervous system becomes more sensitive to alcohol with age.
- Chronic medical conditions worsened by alcohol:
    - Liver diseases (cirrhosis, hepatitis).
    - Gastrointestinal (GI) diseases (GI bleeding, gastric reflux, ulcer).

TABLE 9-2. Alcohol and Medication Interactions

Medication	Result of Concurrent Alcohol Use
H_2 blockers	Higher BALs
Benzodiazepines, tricyclics, narcotics, barbiturates, antihistamines	↑ sedation
Aspirin, NSAIDs	Prolonged bleeding time; Irritation of gastric lining
Metronidazole, sulfonamides, long-acting hypoglycemics	Nausea and vomiting
Reserpine, nitroglycerin, hydralazine	↑ risk of hypotension
Acetaminophen, isoniazid, phenylbutazone	↑ hepatotoxicity
Antihypertensives, antidiabetics, ulcer drugs, gout medications	Worsen underlying disease

- Cardiovascular diseases (hypertension, heart failure).
- Metabolic/endocrine diseases (gout, diabetes).
- Mental disorders (depression, anxiety).
■ Alcohol and medication interactions (see Table 9-2).

Psychiatric Manifestations of Major Neurocognitive Disorders (Dementia)

Behavioral symptoms are quite common in patients with major neurocognitive disorder, and quite often the source of many psychosocial problems surrounding their care. Agitation and aggression can be distressing and dangerous for caregivers, as well as unsafe for patients. Behavioral disinhibition is fairly common in major neurocognitive disorders and causes patients to act in ways that are quite unlike their typical behaviors (stripping off clothes in public, sexualized behavior, cursing).

- Mood disorders:
  - Difficult to diagnose in a patient with confirmed major neurocognitive disorder.
  - Patients with major neurocognitive disorders may display many symptoms of depression that are merely natural manifestations of their disease.
- Aggression:
  - May be provoked by the patient's confusion in the setting of cognitive, memory, and language deficits.
  - May be provoked by hallucinations or delusions.
- Psychosis:
  - Delusions are reported in up to 50% of Alzheimer patients.
  - Hallucinations (mostly auditory and/or visual) can be seen in at least 25% of patients with a major neurocognitive disorder.
  - If hallucinations do not bother the patient or interfere with caring for the patient, pharmacotherapy is unnecessary.

WARDS TIP

Visual hallucinations early in dementia suggest a diagnosis of neurocognitive disorder due to Lewy body disease. Antipsychotics should be avoided as these patients are sensitive to extrapyramidal symptoms (EPS).

TREATMENT

Behavioral and environmental treatments for behavioral symptoms are much preferred in the elderly. Pharmacological methods are appropriate in the setting of potentially harmful behaviors, but care must be taken in dosing, duration of treatment, and interactions with other medications.

- Nonpharmacological treatments:
    - Music, art, exercise, and pet therapy.
    - Strict daily schedules to minimize changes in routine.
    - Continual reorientation of patient.
    - Reduce stimuli (quiet living environments).
    - Surround patient with familiar objects (family photos, a favorite quilt, etc.).
- Pharmacological treatments:
    - Antipsychotics:
        - Limited efficacy and increase in mortality.
        - Try olanzapine (Zyprexa) or quetiapine (Seroquel) in patients with severe symptoms.
        - Can also use short-term haloperidol (Haldol) or risperidone (Risperdal).
    - Anxiolytics:
        - Anxiety symptoms may be due to unrecognized depression and respond well to an SSRI.
        - Reserve benzodiazepines for very short-term, acute episodes and remember to watch for disinhibition (paradoxical agitation).
        - Mood stabilizers: Few studies on their effectiveness in the elderly.

Sleep Disturbance

The incidence of sleep disorders increases with aging. Elderly people often report difficulty sleeping, daytime drowsiness, and daytime napping.

- Outside of normal changes associated with aging (see Table 9-3), causes of sleep disturbances may include other medical conditions, drug/alcohol use, social stressors, and medications.
- Patients with movement disorders (Parkinson disease, progressive supranuclear palsy) have shallow sleep and may be more restless at night because of trouble turning in bed.
- Restless leg movements during sleep, likely due to a dopamine imbalance, are called periodic leg movements (PLMs).

TABLE 9-3. **Normal Sleep Changes in Geriatric Patients**

Rapid eye movement (REM) sleep	↓ REM latency and ↓ total REM
Non-REM sleep	↑ amounts of stage 1 and 2 sleep, ↓ amounts of stage 3 and 4 sleep (deep sleep)
Sleep efficiency	↓ (frequent nocturnal awakenings)
Amount of total sleep	↓
Sleep cycle	Sleep cycle advances (earlier to bed, earlier to rise)

- Nonpharmacological treatment approaches should be tried first (alcohol cessation, increased daily structure, elimination of daytime naps, treatment of underlying medical conditions that may be exacerbating sleep problems).
- Sedative-hypnotic drugs are more likely to cause side effects when used by the elderly (memory impairment, ataxia, paradoxical excitement, and rebound insomnia).
- If sedative-hypnotics must be prescribed, medications such as trazodone are safer than the more sedating benzodiazepines, but be careful of orthostasis.

Other Issues

RESTRAINTS

- In nonemergency situations, restraints should be used as a last resort and the patient should be reassessed at regular intervals.
- Patient safety, health, and well-being should be the most important concern in the matter of restraint use.

MEDICATIONS

- Many older people are on multiple medications ("polypharmacy").
- They suffer from more side effects because of decrease in lean body mass and impaired liver and kidney function.
- When confronted with a new symptom in an elderly patient on multiple medications, always try to remove a medication before adding one.

ELDER ABUSE

- Types: Physical abuse, psychological abuse (threats, insults, etc.), neglect (withholding of care), exploitation (misuse of finances), and rarely sexual abuse.
- Approximately 10% of all people more than 65 years old; underreported by victims.
- Perpetrator is usually a caregiver (spouse or adult child) who lives with the victim.
- Physicians are mandated to report suspected elder abuse.

NURSING HOMES

- Provide care and rehabilitation for chronically ill and impaired patients as well as for patients who are in need of short-term care before returning to their prior living arrangements.
- The majority of patients stay permanently, and fewer than half are discharged after only a short period of time.

CHAPTER 10

PSYCHIATRIC DISORDERS IN CHILDREN

Psychiatric Examination of a Child	120
Sources of Information	120
Methods of Gathering Information	120
Safety Assessment	120
Intellectual Disability	120
Diagnosis and DSM-5 Criteria	120
Epidemiology	121
Etiology	121
Global Developmental Delay	121
Specific Learning Disorder (LD)	122
Diagnosis and DSM-5 Criteria	122
Epidemiology	122
Etiology	122
Comorbidity	122
Treatment	122
Communication Disorders	122
Treatment	123
Attention Deficit/Hyperactivity Disorder (ADHD)	123
Diagnosis and DSM-5 Criteria	123
Epidemiology	124
Etiology	124
Course/Prognosis	124
Treatment	124
Autism Spectrum Disorder (ASD)	125
Diagnosis and DSM-5 Criteria	125
Epidemiology	125
Etiology	125
Prognosis and Treatment	126
Tic Disorders	126
Tourette's Disorder	126
Disruptive and Conduct Disorders	127
Oppositional Defiant Disorder (ODD)	127
Conduct Disorder	128
Elimination Disorders	129
DSM-5 Diagnosis	129
Epidemiology	129
Etiology	129
Treatment	129
Child Abuse	130
Physical Abuse	130
Sexual Abuse	130
Psychological Abuse	130
Neglect	131
Treatment	131
Sequelae	131

Psychiatric Examination of a Child

SOURCES OF INFORMATION

Gather and integrate collateral information from multiple sources to obtain as accurate a clinical picture as possible: primary caregivers, teachers, pediatricians, and the child welfare system (if relevant).

METHODS OF GATHERING INFORMATION

Determine the child's **developmental stage** and tailor the interview appropriately.

- **Play therapy:** Utilizes the child's *symbolic play, storytelling,* or drawing as a forum for expression of emotions and experiences.
- **Classroom observation:** A window into the child's functioning in school.
- **Formal neuropsychological testing:** Quantitatively assesses a child's strengths and weaknesses by examination of cognitive profile: intelligence quotient (IQ); language and visual-motor skills; memory, attention, and organizational abilities.
- **Kaufman Assessment Battery for Children (K-ABC):** Intelligence test comparing intellectual capacity with acquired knowledge of patients between 2 and 12 years old.
- **Wechsler Intelligence Scale for Children-Revised (WISC-R):** Assesses verbal, performance, and full-scale IQ of patients between 6 and 16 years old.

SAFETY ASSESSMENT

 WARDS TIP

Asking about suicide can be preventive, not causal.

- Always screen for safety (e.g., suicidal/homicidal ideation and psychotic thoughts, particularly command auditory hallucinations) in a developmentally appropriate manner. Also screen for self-injurious behavior as this may indicate an increased risk for suicidal behavior.
- In the United States, suicide is the third leading cause of death in children 10–14 years old and the second leading cause of death in individuals ages 15–24.

Intellectual Disability

Intellectual disability (intellectual developmental disorder) replaces the term mental retardation (MR) as per U.S. law (Rosa's law), with the intention of decreasing stigmatization. Intellectual disability (ID) is characterized by impaired cognitive and adaptive/social functioning. Severity level is currently based on adaptive functioning, indicating the degree of support required. A single IQ score does not adequately capture this and is no longer used solely to determine ID severity.

DIAGNOSIS AND DSM-5 CRITERIA

- **Deficits in intellectual functioning,** such as reasoning, problem solving, planning, abstract thinking, judgment, and learning.
- **Deficits in adaptive functioning,** such as communication, social participation, and independent living.

- Deficits affect multiple domains: conceptual, practical, and social.
- Onset occurs during the developmental period.
- Intellectual deficits are confirmed by clinical assessment and standardized intelligence testing (scores at least two standard deviations below the population mean).
- Adaptive functioning deficits require ongoing support for activities of daily life.
- Severity levels: mild, moderate, severe, and profound.

EPIDEMIOLOGY

- Overall: 1% of population.
- Severe ID: 6/1000.

ETIOLOGY

- Causes include genetic, prenatal, perinatal, and postnatal conditions (see Table 10-1).
- Fifty percent of ID cases have no identifiable cause.

Global Developmental Delay

- Failure to meet expected developmental milestones in several areas of intellectual functioning.
- Diagnosis reserved for patients less than 5 years old when severity level cannot be reliably assessed via standardized testing. Patients will need to be reevaluated in the future to clarify the diagnosis.

WARDS TIP

Characteristic physical features of genetic syndromes:
- Down syndrome: Epicanthic folds, flat nasal bridge, and palmar crease
- Fragile X syndrome: Macrocephaly, joint hyperlaxity, and macroorchidism in postpubertal males.
- Prader–Willi syndrome: Obese, small stature, and almond-shaped eyes.

KEY FACT

Fragile X Syndrome Facts and Stats
- Most common inherited form of ID.
- Second most common cause of ID.
- Due to *FMR*-1 gene mutation.
- Males > females.

KEY FACT

Down Syndrome Facts and Stats
- 1/700 live births.
- Most common chromosomal disorder.
- Trisomy 21 = 3 copies of chromosome 21.

TABLE 10-1. Causes of Intellectual Disability

Cause	Examples
Genetic	- **Down syndrome:** Trisomy 21 (1/700 live births) - **Fragile X syndrome:** Involves mutation of X chromosome, second most common cause of intellectual disability, males > females - *Others:* Phenylketonuria, familial mental retardation, Prader–Willi syndrome, Williams syndrome, Angelman syndrome, tuberous sclerosis
Prenatal	Infection and toxins (**TORCH**): - **T**oxoplasmosis - **O**ther (syphilis, AIDS, alcohol/illicit drugs) - **R**ubella (German measles) - **C**ytomegalovirus (CMV) - **H**erpes simplex
Perinatal	Anoxia, prematurity, birth trauma, meningitis, hyperbilirubinemia
Postnatal	Hypothyroidism, malnutrition, toxin exposure, trauma

KEY FACT

<u>Fetal Alcohol Exposure Facts</u>
Fetal Alcohol Syndrome (FAS) = Leading *preventable* cause of birth defects and ID.

Three features of FAS:
1. Growth retardation
2. CNS involvement (structural, neurologic, functional)
3. Facial dysmorphology (smooth philtrum, short palpebral fissures, thin vermillion border)

Fetal Alcohol Spectrum Disorders

Fetal alcohol exposure of any amount may cause a range of developmental disabilities, which are often under-recognized.

WARDS TIP

Always rule out sensory deficits before diagnosing a specific learning disorder.

Specific Learning Disorder (LD)

Characterized by delayed cognitive development in a particular academic domain.

DIAGNOSIS AND DSM-5 CRITERIA

- Significantly impaired academic skills which are below expectation for chronological age and interfere with academics, occupation, or activities of daily living (ADLs).
- Begins during school but may become more impairing as demands increase.
- Affected areas: reading (e.g., dyslexia), writing, or arithmetic (e.g., dyscalculia).
- Not better accounted for by intellectual disabilities, visual/auditory deficits, language barriers, or subpar education.

EPIDEMIOLOGY

- Prevalence in school age children: 5–15%.
- Males > females affected.

ETIOLOGY

- Environmental factors: Increased risk with prematurity, very low birth weight, and prenatal nicotine exposure.
- Genetic factors: Increased risk in first-degree relatives of affected individuals.

COMORBIDITY

- Commonly co-occurs with other neurodevelopmental disorders, such as ADHD, communication disorders, developmental coordination disorder, and autistic spectrum disorder (ASD).
- Comorbid with other mental disorders, including anxiety, depressive, and bipolar disorders.

TREATMENT

- Systematic, individualized education tailored to child's specific needs.
- Behavioral techniques may be used to improve learning skills.

Communication Disorders

Communication disorder includes impaired speech, language or social communication that are below expectation for chronological age, begin in the early developmental period, and lead to academic or adaptive issues.

- Language disorder—difficulty acquiring and using language due to expressive and/or receptive impairment (e.g., reduced vocabulary, limited sentence structure, impairments in discourse). Increased risk in families of affected individuals.
- Speech sound disorder (phonological disorder)—difficulty producing articulate, intelligible speech.

- Childhood-onset fluency disorder (stuttering)—dysfluency and speech motor production issues. Increased risk of stuttering in first-degree relatives of affected individuals.
- Social (pragmatic) communication disorder—challenges with the social use of verbal and nonverbal communication. If restricted/repetitive behaviors, activities, or interests are also present, consider diagnosis of ASD. Increased risk with family history of communication disorders, ASD, or specific learning disorder.

TREATMENT

- Speech and language therapy, family counseling.
- Tailor educational supports to meet the individual's needs.

 A 10-year-old girl is referred for psychiatric evaluation because of academic and behavior problems at school over the last year. In the office, she is constantly on the move and appears to be "driven by a motor." During the interview, she has difficulty staying focused on the questions. Her mother complains that she never seems to pay attention. Her teacher reports that the patient does not follow directions. She has trouble waiting her turn and often blurts out answers during class. Although she seems to comprehend the material, she makes careless mistakes on homework and tests.

What is the most likely diagnosis?

The patient has classic symptoms of attention deficit/hyperactivity disorder (ADHD) with both inattention and hyperactivity occurring in two different settings (home and school).

What treatment is indicated?

If the child does not have any contraindications, stimulant medications are the first-line treatment for ADHD.

Attention Deficit/Hyperactivity Disorder (ADHD)

ADHD is characterized by persistent **inattention**, **hyperactivity**, and **impulsivity** inconsistent with the patient's developmental stage. There are three subcategories of ADHD: predominantly inattentive type, predominantly hyperactive/impulsive type, and combined type.

DIAGNOSIS AND DSM-5 CRITERIA

- Two symptom domains: inattentiveness and hyperactivity/impulsivity.
- At least six inattentive symptoms:
  - Does not pay attention to details or makes careless mistakes.
  - Has difficulty sustaining attention.
  - Does not appear to listen.
  - Struggles to follow instructions.
  - Unorganized.

- Avoids or dislikes tasks requiring high cognitive demands.
- Misplaces or loses objects frequently.
- Easily distracted.
- Forgetful in daily activities.

and/or

- At least six hyperactivity/impulsivity symptoms:
  - Fidgets with hands/feet or squirms in chair.
  - Has difficulty remaining seated.
  - Runs about or climbs excessively in childhood (extreme restlessness in adults).
  - Difficulty engaging in activities quietly.
  - Acts as if driven by a motor (may be an internal sensation in adults).
  - Talks excessively.
  - Blurts out answers before questions have been completed.
  - Difficulty waiting or taking turns.
  - Interrupts or intrudes upon others.
- Symptoms more than 6 months and present in **two** or more settings (e.g., home, school, work).
- Symptoms interfere with or reduce quality of social/academic/occupational functioning.
- Onset **prior to age 12,** but can be diagnosed retrospectively in adulthood.
- Symptoms not due to another mental disorder.

EPIDEMIOLOGY

- Prevalence: 5% of children and 2.5% of adults.
- Males > females with 2:1 ratio.
- Females present more often with inattentive symptoms.

ETIOLOGY

The etiology of ADHD is multifactorial and may include:

- Genetic factors: Increased rate in first-degree relatives of affected individuals.
- Environmental factors: Low birth weight, smoking during pregnancy, childhood abuse/neglect, neurotoxin/alcohol exposure.

COURSE/PROGNOSIS

- Stable through adolescence.
- Many continue to have symptoms as adults (inattentive > hyperactive).
- High incidence of comorbid oppositional defiant disorder, conduct disorder (CD), and specific learning disorder.

> **KEY FACT**
>
> Stimulants are first-line treatment in ADHD.

TREATMENT

Multimodal treatment plan: Medications are the most effective treatment for decreasing core symptoms, but should be used in conjunction with educational and behavioral interventions.

- Pharmacological treatments:
  - First-line: Stimulants e.g., methylphenidate compounds, dextroamphetamine, and mixed amphetamine salts.

- Second-line choice: Atomoxetine, a norepinephrine reuptake inhibitor.
- Alpha-2 agonists (e.g., clonidine, **guanfacine**) can be used instead of or as adjunctive therapy to stimulants.
- Nonpharmacological treatments:
  - Behavior modification techniques and social skills training.
  - Educational interventions (i.e., classroom modifications).
  - Parental psychoeducation.

Autism Spectrum Disorder (ASD)

ASD is characterized by impairments in **social communication/interaction** and **restrictive, repetitive behaviors/interests**. This disorder encompasses the spectrum of symptomatology formerly diagnosed as autism, Asperger's disorder, childhood disintegrative disorder, and pervasive developmental disorder.

DIAGNOSIS AND DSM-5 CRITERIA

- **Problems with social interaction and communication:**
  - Impaired social/emotional reciprocity (e.g., inability to hold conversations).
  - Deficits in nonverbal communication skills (e.g., decreased eye contact).
  - Interpersonal/relational challenges (e.g., lack of interest in peers).
- **Restricted, repetitive patterns of behavior, interests, and activities:**
  - Intense, peculiar interests (e.g., preoccupation with unusual objects).
  - Inflexible adherence to rituals (e.g., rigid thought patterns).
  - Stereotyped, repetitive motor mannerisms (e.g., hand flapping).
  - Hyperreactivity/hyporeactivity to sensory input (e.g., hypersensitive to particular textures).
- Abnormalities in functioning begin in the early developmental period.
- Not better accounted for by ID or global developmental delay. When ID and ASD co-occur, social communication is below expectation based on developmental level.
- Causes significant social or occupational impairment.

WARDS TIP

Consider ASD as the diagnosis if there is a rapid deterioration of social and/or language skills during the first 2 years of life.

Complete an appropriate workup, such as auditory testing, prior to diagnosing ASD.

If skills are lost after age 2 or more expansive losses occur (e.g., self-care, motor skills), an extensive medical workup needs to be initiated.

EPIDEMIOLOGY

- Recent increase in prevalence to one percent of population. Could be related to expansion of diagnostic classification and/or increased awareness/recognition.
- The 4:1 ratio of diagnosis in males:females.
- Symptoms typically recognized between 12 and 24 months old, but varies based on severity.

WARDS TIP

Assess for a potential cause of pain/discomfort if a nonverbal ASD patient presents with new onset aggression or self-injurious behavior.

ETIOLOGY

Etiology of ASD is multifactorial:

- Prenatal neurological insults (e.g., infections, drugs), advanced paternal age, and low birth weight.
- Fifteen percent of ASD cases are associated with a known genetic mutation.
- Fragile X syndrome = most common known single gene cause of ASD.

- Other genetic causes of ASD: Down syndrome, Rett syndrome, tuberous sclerosis.
- High comorbidity with ID.
- Association with epilepsy.

PROGNOSIS AND TREATMENT

ASD is a chronic condition. The prognosis is variable, but the two most important predictors of adult outcome are level of intellectual functioning and language impairment. Only a minority of patients can live and work independently in adulthood. There is no cure for autism, but various treatments are used to help manage symptoms and improve basic social, communicative, and cognitive skills:

- Early intervention.
- Remedial education.
- Behavioral therapy.
- Psychoeducation.
- Low-dose atypical antipsychotic medications (e.g., risperidone, aripiprazole) may help reduce disruptive behavior, aggression, and irritability.

Tic Disorders

TOURETTE'S DISORDER

Tics are defined as sudden, rapid, repetitive, stereotyped movements or vocalizations. Although experienced as involuntary, patients can learn to temporarily suppress tics. Prior to the tic, patients may feel a premonitory urge (somatic sensation), with subsequent tension release after the tic. Anxiety, excitement, and fatigue can be aggravating factors for tics. Tics may present as simple or complex, depending on length of time, purpose, and orchestration.

Tourette's disorder is the **most severe** of the tic disorders. It is characterized by **multiple motor tics and at least one vocal tic lasting for at least 1 year**. Vocal tics may appear many years after the motor tics, and they may wax and wane in frequency. The most common **motor tics** involve the face and head, such as eye blinking and throat clearing.

Examples of **vocal tics**:

- *Coprolalia*—utterance of obscene, taboo words as an abrupt, sharp bark or grunt.
- *Echolalia*—repeating others' words.

Diagnosis and DSM-5 Criteria

- Multiple motor and at least 1 vocal tics present (not required to occur concurrently) for more than 1 year since onset of first tic.
- Onset prior to age 18 years.
- Not caused by a substance (e.g., cocaine) or another medical condition (e.g., Huntington disease).

Epidemiology

- Transient tic behaviors: common in children.
- Tourette's disorder: 3 per 1000 school-age children.
- Prevalence: boys > girls.

WARDS TIP

Tic disorders are one of the few psychiatric disorders in which diagnostic criteria do not require symptoms to cause significant distress.

Etiology
- Genetic factors: >55% concordance rate in monozygotic twins.
- Prenatal/perinatal factors: Older paternal age, obstetrical complications, maternal smoking, and low birth weight.
- Psychological factors: Symptom exacerbations with stressful life events.

Course/Prognosis
- Onset typically occurs between 4 and 6 years, with the peak severity between ages 10 and 12.
- Tics wax and wane and change in type.
- Symptoms tend to decrease in adolescence and significantly diminish in adulthood.
- High comorbidity with OCD, ADHD, LD, and ASD.

Treatment
- Psychoeducation.
- **Behavioral interventions**—habit reversal therapy.
- Medications—utilize only if tics become severely impairing or also treating comorbidities. Due to the fluctuating course of the disorder, it can be difficult to determine medication efficacy.
- **Alpha-2 agonists: guanfacine (first choice)**, clonidine (more sedating).
- In severe cases, can consider treatment with atypical (e.g., risperidone) or typical antipsychotics (e.g., pimozide).

Other tic disorders include:

- **Persistent (chronic) motor or vocal tic disorder**: Single or multiple motor or vocal tics (but not both) that have never met criteria for Tourette's.
- **Provisional tic disorder**: Single or multiple motor and/or vocal tics less than 1 year that have never met criteria for Tourette's.

Disruptive and Conduct Disorders

These disorders involve **problematic interactions** or **inflicting harm** on others. While disruptive behaviors may appear within the scope of normal development, they become pathologic when the frequency, pervasiveness, and severity impair functioning of the individual or others.

OPPOSITIONAL DEFIANT DISORDER (ODD)

A maladaptive pattern of **irritability/anger, defiance, or vindictiveness**, which causes dysfunction, or distress in the patient or those affected. These interpersonal difficulties involve at least one non-sibling.

Diagnosis and DSM-5 Criteria
Characterized by at least four symptoms present for more than or equal to 6 months (with at least one individual who is not a sibling):

- **Anger/Irritable mood**—loses temper frequently; often angry and resentful.
- **Argumentative/Defiant behavior**—breaks rules, blames others, argues with authority figures, and deliberately aggravates others.

WARDS TIP

A child may have **oppositional defiant disorder** if he/she has no difficulty getting along with peers but will not comply with rules from parents or teachers.

KEY FACT

Unlike conduct disorder, ODD does *not* involve physical aggression or violating the basic rights of others.

- **Vindictiveness**—spiteful/vindictive at least two times in the past 6 months.
- Behaviors are associated with distress in the individual or others, or negatively impact functioning.
- Behaviors do not occur exclusively during another mental disorder.

Epidemiology

- Prevalence: Approximately 3%.
- Onset usually during preschool years: Seen more often in boys before adolescence.
- Increased incidence of comorbid substance use and ADHD.
- Although ODD often precedes CD, most do not develop CD.

Treatment

- **Behavior modification**, conflict management training, and improving problem-solving skills.
- Parent Management Training (PMT) can help with setting limits and enforcing consistent rules.
- Medications are used to treat comorbid conditions, such as ADHD.

> **KEY FACT**
>
> **C**ruelty to animals may be indicative of **C**onduct disorder.

CONDUCT DISORDER

CD includes the most serious disruptive behaviors, which **violate the rights of other humans and animals**. These individuals inflict cruelty and harm through physical and sexual violence. They may **lack remorse** for committing crimes or **lack empathy** for their victims.

Diagnosis and DSM-5 Criteria

A pattern of **recurrently violating the basic rights of others or societal norms.** The individual has displayed at least three of the following behaviors exhibited over the last year and at least one occurring within the past 6 months:

- **Aggression to people and animals:** Bullies/threatens/intimidates others; initiation of physical aggression, including use of a weapon; rape; cruelty to animals; robbery.
- **Destruction of property** (e.g., fire setting).
- **Deceitfulness or theft:** Burglary; lying to obtain goods/favors.
- **Serious violations of rules:** Runs away from home, stays out late at night, and often truant from school before age 13 years old.

> **KEY FACT**
>
> Male versus Female Misconduct
>
> **Males:** Higher risk of fighting, stealing, fire-setting, and vandalism.
>
> **Females:** Higher risk of lying, running away, prostitution, and substance use.

Epidemiology

- Lifetime prevalence: 9%.
- More common in males.
- High incidence of comorbid ADHD and ODD.
- Associated with antisocial personality disorder.

Treatment

- A multimodal treatment approach with **behavior modification**, family, and community involvement.
- PMT can help parents with limit setting and enforcing consistent rules.
- Medications can be used to target comorbid symptoms and aggression (e.g., SSRIs, guanfacine, propranolol, mood stabilizers, antipsychotics).

> **KEY FACT**
>
> Alcohol is the most common drug of abuse by adolescents, followed by cannabis.

Elimination Disorders

Characterized by **developmentally inappropriate elimination of urine or feces**. Though typically involuntary, this may be intentional. The course may be *primary* (never established continence) or *secondary* (continence achieved for a period and then lost). Incontinence can cause significant distress or impair social or other areas of functioning.

DSM-5 DIAGNOSIS

Enuresis:

- **Recurrent urination into clothes or bed-wetting.**
- Occurs two times per week for at least 3 consecutive months or results in clinical distress or marked impairment.
- At least 5 years old developmentally.
- Can occur during sleep (**nocturnal**), waking hours (**diurnal**), or both.
- Not due to a substance (e.g., diuretic) or another medical condition (e.g., urinary tract infection, neurogenic bladder, diabetes).

Encopresis:

- **Recurrent defecation into inappropriate places** (e.g., clothes, floor).
- Occurs at least one time per month for at least 3 months.
- At least 4 years old developmentally.
- Not due to a substance (e.g., laxatives) or another medical condition (e.g., hypothyroidism, anal fissure, spina bifida) except via a constipation-related mechanism.

EPIDEMIOLOGY

- Prevalence of enuresis decreases with age:
    - 5–10% of 5 year olds; 3–5% of 10 year olds; 1% of > 15 year olds.
    - Nocturnal enuresis more common in boys; diurnal enuresis more common in girls.
- Prevalence of encopresis: 1% of 5-year-old children; boys > girls.

ETIOLOGY

- Genetic predisposition for nocturnal enuresis:
    - About four times increased risk if history of maternal urinary incontinence.
    - About 10 times increased risk if history of paternal urinary incontinence.
- Psychosocial stressors may contribute to secondary incontinence.
- Encopresis: often related to constipation/impaction with overflow incontinence.

WARDS TIP

The majority of enuresis cases spontaneously remit (5–10% per year) by adolescence.

TREATMENT

- **Psychoeducation** is key for children and their primary caregivers; provide information about high spontaneous remission rates.
- Only treat if symptoms are distressing and impairing. Engage the patient as an active participant in the treatment plan. Encourage investment in a waterproof mattress.
- Parent management treatment (PMT) for managing intentional elimination.

- **Enuresis treatment:**
  - Limit fluid intake and caffeine at night.
  - Behavioral program with monitoring and reward system, "bladder training" exercises, or **urine alarm** (upgrade from the **"bell and pad" method**).
  - Pharmacology can be used if the above methods are ineffective or for diurnal enuresis.
    - **Desmopressin (DDAVP)**, an antidiuretic hormone analogue, is the **first-line medication**.
    - **Imipramine**, a tricyclic antidepressant, can be used at low doses for refractory cases but has less tolerable side effects.
- **Encopresis without constipation:** Comprehensive behavioral program ("bowel retraining") for appropriate elimination.
- **Encopresis due to constipation:** Initial bowel cleaning followed by stool softeners, high-fiber diet, and toileting routine in conjunction with a behavioral program.

Child Abuse

Child abuse encompasses **physical** abuse, **sexual** abuse, **emotional** abuse, and **neglect. Toxic stress** may result when children **endure prolonged, severe trauma and adversity** without the buffer of supportive caregivers. This can disrupt a child's development and lead to a spectrum of pathologic sequelae.

- About **1 million** cases of **child maltreatment** in the United States.
- Up to 2,500 deaths per year caused by abuse in the United States.

These numbers may be an underestimation as many cases go undetected and unreported.

PHYSICAL ABUSE

- Any act that results in non-accidental injury and may be the result of severe corporal punishment committed by an individual responsible for the child.
- Physical exam and x-rays may demonstrate multiple, concerning injuries not consistent with child's developmental age.
- Most common perpetrator is a first-degree male caregiver (e.g., parent, guardian, mother's partner).

SEXUAL ABUSE

- Any sexual act involving a child intended to provide sexual gratification to an individual responsible for the child.
- Sexual abuse is the most invasive form of abuse and results in detrimental lifetime effects on victim.
- Data indicates approximately 25% of girls and 9% of boys are exposed to sexual abuse. Abuse is generally underreported and males are less likely than females to report it.
- Children are most at risk of sexual abuse during preadolescence.

PSYCHOLOGICAL ABUSE

Non-accidental verbal or symbolic acts that result in psychological damage.

WARDS TIP

- Red flags for physical abuse: delayed medical care for injury, inconsistent explanation of injury, multiple injuries in various stages of healing, spiral bone fractures, bruising patterns consistent with hand/belt, cigarette burns, and head injuries.
- Red flags for sexual abuse: sexually transmitted diseases, recurrent urinary tract infections, prepubertal vaginal bleeding, pregnancy, or trauma/bruising/inflammation of genitals or anus.

WARDS TIP

If a child reports sexual abuse, it should be taken seriously as it is rarely unfounded.

NEGLECT

- Failure to provide a child with adequate food, shelter, supervision, medical care, education, and/or affection.
- Victims of neglect may exhibit poor hygiene, malnutrition, stunted growth, developmental delays, and failure to thrive.
- Severe deprivation can result in death, particularly in infants.
- Neglect accounts for the majority of cases reported to child protection services.

TREATMENT

Early intervention can potentially mitigate the negative sequelae and facilitate recovery.

SEQUELAE

- Increased risk of developing posttraumatic stress disorder, anxiety disorders, depressive disorders, dissociative disorders, self-destructive behaviors, and substance use disorders.
- Increased risk of continuing intergenerational abuse cycle with partners and children.

WARDS TIP

Doctors are *mandated reporters*, thus legally required to report all cases of suspected child abuse to the appropriate social service agencies.

CHAPTER 11

DISSOCIATIVE DISORDERS

Dissociative Amnesia	134
Diagnosis and DSM-5 Criteria	134
Epidemiology/Etiology	134
Treatment	134
Depersonalization/Derealization Disorder	135
Diagnosis and DSM-5 Criteria	135
Epidemiology/Etiology	135
Course and Prognosis	135
Treatment	135
Dissociative Identity Disorder (Multiple Personality Disorder)	136
Diagnosis and DSM-5 Criteria	136
Epidemiology/Etiology	136
Course and Prognosis	136
Treatment	136
Other Specified Dissociative Disorder	137
DSM-5 examples	137

Dissociation can be understood as a **disruption in the integrated sense of self**. This may involve **lapses in autobiographical memory** (*amnesia*) and **feelings of detachment from one's self** (*depersonalization*) or from one's surroundings (*derealization*). These symptoms often develop in the context or aftermath of **significant trauma**, particularly **during childhood**. Dissociation may initially help buffer the impact of a trauma, but can also become pathological and maladaptive. While the dissociative disorders are closely related to the stressor- and trauma-related disorders, they are classified separately in the DSM-5.

WARDS TIP

Dissociative responses typically occur during stressful and traumatic events.

KEY FACT

Dissociative amnesia refers to disruption in the continuity of an individual's memory. Patients with dissociative amnesia report gaps in the recollection of particular events, usually traumatic ones.

Dissociative Amnesia

Individuals with dissociative amnesia are unable to remember important personal information or history, often **traumatic** in nature. **Procedural memory is preserved**, distinguishing dissociative amnesia from other conditions resulting in memory loss (e.g., major neurocognitive disorders/dementias). The unrecalled autobiographical information has been stored in memory and is thus potentially retrievable. Dissociative amnesia rarely generalizes to encompass complete memory loss. More commonly, a single period of time (*localized amnesia*) or certain events (*selective amnesia*) are forgotten. Affected individuals often do not have insight regarding their deficits. There is a significant incidence of comorbid major depressive disorder or persistent depressive disorder (dysthymia) and an **increased risk for suicide**—particularly as amnesia resolves and the overwhelming memories return.

WARDS TIP

Patients suffering from dissociative amnesia can experience periods of flashbacks, nightmares, or behavioral reenactments of their trauma.

KEY FACT

Although dissociative fugue is now considered a subtype of dissociative amnesia disorder, it more commonly occurs with dissociative identity disorder.

DIAGNOSIS AND DSM-5 CRITERIA

- An inability to recall important autobiographical information, usually involving a traumatic or stressful event, that is inconsistent with ordinary forgetfulness.
- May present with *dissociative fugue*: **sudden, unexpected travel away from home**, accompanied by amnesia for identity or other autobiographical information.
- Not due to the physiological effects of a substance or another medical/psychiatric/neurological disorder (including traumatic brain injury).
- Symptoms cause significant distress or impairment in daily functioning.

EPIDEMIOLOGY/ETIOLOGY

- Lifetime prevalence is 6–7%.
- More common in women than men.
- Single or repeated traumas often occur prior to the development of amnesia.

KEY FACT

Abreaction is the strong emotional reaction patients may experience when retrieving traumatic memories.

TREATMENT

- Important to establish the patient's safety.
- Psychotherapy (e.g., supportive, CBT, hypnosis) is the mainstay of treatment.
- No medications have demonstrated efficacy in dissociative amnesia.

WARDS TIP

Fugue: Think of a *forget*ful *fug*itive who runs away and forms a new identity.

A 19-year-old man is found wandering several miles from home 3 days after a missing persons report was filed by his family. He cannot recall his full name or address, even when shown his ID card. His family reports that he recently returned from combat deployment.

Likely diagnosis?

Dissociative amnesia with dissociative fugue

Depersonalization/Derealization Disorder

Characterized by repeated experiences of **detachment from one's self or surroundings**. Patients may feel as though they are observing themselves from a distance or have an **"out-of-body" experience** (*depersonalization*). They may experience the world around them as though they were **in a dream or movie** (*derealization*).

DIAGNOSIS AND DSM-5 CRITERIA

- Persistent or recurrent experiences of one or both:
  - Depersonalization—experiences of unreality or detachment from one's body, thoughts, feelings, or actions
  - Derealization—experiences of unreality or detachment from one's surroundings.
- Reality testing remains intact during an episode.
- The symptoms cause significant distress or social/occupational impairment.
- Not accounted for by a substance (e.g., drug of abuse, medication), another medical condition, or another mental disorder.

 KEY FACT

Transient experiences of depersonalization or derealization commonly occur in many individuals during times of stress.

EPIDEMIOLOGY/ETIOLOGY

- Lifetime prevalence is 2%.
- Gender ratio 1:1.
- Mean age of onset about 16 years.
- Increased incidence of comorbid anxiety disorders and major depression.
- Severe stress or traumas are predisposing factors.

COURSE AND PROGNOSIS

Often persistent but may wax and wane.

TREATMENT

- Psychodynamic, cognitive-behavioral, hypnotherapy, and supportive therapies may be helpful.
- Lack of evidence for use of medications to treat depersonalization/derealization disorder.

Dissociative Identity Disorder (Multiple Personality Disorder)

Dissociative identity disorder (DID) is characterized by the presence of **more than one distinct personality state** as a result of a fragmented sense of self. DID encompasses features of the other dissociative disorders, such as **amnesia**, **depersonalization**, and **derealization**. DID predominantly develops in **victims of significant and chronic childhood trauma**. Patients diagnosed with DID often cope with posttraumatic stress disorder (PTSD), depression, and suicidality.

DIAGNOSIS AND DSM-5 CRITERIA

- **Disruption of identity** manifested **as two or more distinct personality states** dominating at different times. These symptoms may be observed by others or self-reported.
- **Extensive memory lapses** in autobiographical information, daily occurrences, and/or traumatic events.
- Not due to effects of a substance (drug or medication) or another medical condition.
- The condition causes significant distress or impairment in social/occupational functioning.

EPIDEMIOLOGY/ETIOLOGY

- Rare. No epidemiologic studies of the national prevalence, although a few community-based studies claim a prevalence of 1%.
- Increased prevalence in women versus men.
- A history of childhood physical/sexual abuse or neglect is present in 90% of patients with DID.
- May manifest at any age, but some symptoms are usually present in childhood.
- High incidence of comorbid PTSD, major depression, eating disorders, borderline personality disorder, and substance use disorders.
- More than 70% of patients attempt suicide, often with frequent attempts and self-mutilation.

WARDS TIP

Symptoms of DID may be similar to those seen in borderline personality disorder or psychotic disorders.

COURSE AND PROGNOSIS

- Course is fluctuating but chronic.
- Worst prognosis of all dissociative disorders.

TREATMENT

- Psychotherapy is the standard treatment. Goals include maintenance of safety, stabilization, identity integration, and symptom reduction by working directly with traumatic memories.
- Pharmacotherapy: SSRIs to target comorbid depressive and/or PTSD symptoms (especially hyperarousal). Prazosin may ameliorate nightmares and naltrexone may reduce self-mutilation.

> A 21-year-old woman is brought to the clinic by her boyfriend for evaluation of "memory issues." The patient recently visited her family for the holidays. The boyfriend states that "she had to deal with her abusive, alcoholic father. She seems like someone else ever since." The patient speaks in a childlike singsong voice and asks to be called by a name different than what is listed on her driver's license. She denies any concerns.
>
> ***Most likely diagnosis?***
>
> Dissociative Identity Disorder (DID)

Other Specified Dissociative Disorder

Characterized by symptoms of dissociation that cause significant distress or impairment of functioning, but do not meet the full criteria for a specific dissociative disorder.

DSM-5 EXAMPLES

- Identity disturbance due to prolonged and intense coercive persuasion (e.g., brainwashing, torture, cults).
- Chronic and recurrent syndromes of mixed dissociative symptoms (without dissociative amnesia).
- Dissociative trance: An acute narrowing or loss of awareness of surroundings manifesting as unresponsiveness, potentially with minor stereotyped behaviors (not part of a cultural or religious practice).
- Acute dissociative reactions to stressful events (lasting hours/days → 1 month).

CHAPTER 12

SOMATIC SYMPTOM AND FACTITIOUS DISORDERS

Somatic Symptom Disorder	141
DIAGNOSIS AND DSM-5 CRITERIA	141
EPIDEMIOLOGY	141
TREATMENT AND PROGNOSIS	141
Conversion Disorder (Functional Neurological Symptom Disorder)	141
DIAGNOSIS AND DSM-5 CRITERIA	141
EPIDEMIOLOGY	142
TREATMENT AND PROGNOSIS	142
Illness Anxiety Disorder	142
DIAGNOSIS AND DSM-5 CRITERIA	142
EPIDEMIOLOGY	142
TREATMENT	142
PROGNOSIS	142
Psychological Factors Affecting Other Medical Conditions	143
DIAGNOSIS AND DSM-5 CRITERIA	143
EPIDEMIOLOGY	143
TREATMENT AND PROGNOSIS	143
Factitious Disorder	143
DIAGNOSIS AND DSM-5 CRITERIA	143
EPIDEMIOLOGY	144
TREATMENT AND PROGNOSIS	144
Malingering	144
PRESENTATION	144
EPIDEMIOLOGY	145
MANAGEMENT	145
Review of Distinguishing Features	145

Patients with somatic symptom disorders present with prominent physical symptoms associated with significant distress or impairment in social, occupational, or other areas of functioning. While these patients may or may not have an associated medical condition, their focus is on their distressing somatic symptoms as well as their thoughts, feelings, and behaviors in response to these symptoms.

- Types of somatic symptom and related disorders include:
  - Somatic symptom disorder.
  - Conversion disorder (functional neurological symptom disorder).
  - Illness anxiety disorder.
  - Psychological factors affecting other medical conditions.
  - Factitious disorder.
  - Other specified somatic symptom and related disorder.
  - Unspecified somatic symptom and related disorder.

Up to 30% of primary care patients present with medically unexplained symptoms. In many cases, unspoken psychological needs manifest as physical symptoms. The symptoms may not make physiological "sense" but rather follow the patient's conception of how their body works.

> Ms. Thomas is a 31-year-old woman who was referred to a psychiatrist by her gynecologist after undergoing multiple exploratory surgeries for abdominal pain and gynecologic concerns with no definitive findings. The patient reports that she has had extensive medical problems dating back to adolescence. She reports periods of extreme abdominal pain, vomiting, diarrhea, and possible food intolerances. The obstetrician is her fourth provider because "my other doctors were not able to help me." Ms. Thomas reports fear that her current physician will also fail to relieve her distress. She was reluctant to see a psychiatrist and did so only after her obstetrician agreed to follow her after her psychiatric appointment.
>
> Ms. Thomas states that her problems worsened in college, which was the first time she underwent surgery. She reports that due to her health problems and severe lack of energy, it took her 5½ years to graduate from college. She did better for a year or two after college but then had a return of symptoms. She reports recently feeling very lonely and isolated because she has not been able to find a boyfriend who can tolerate her frequent illnesses. She also reports that physical intimacy is difficult for her because she finds sex painful. Additionally, she is concerned that she might lose her job due to the number of days she has missed from work due to her abdominal pain, fatigue, and weakness.
>
> ### What is the diagnosis?
>
> *Somatic symptom disorder.* Ms. Thomas has a history of multiple somatic complaints lasting at least 6 months, along with a high level of anxiety about her symptoms and excessive time and energy devoted to her health concerns. She has had multiple medical procedures and significant impairment in her social and occupational functioning.

Somatic Symptom Disorder

Patients with somatic symptom disorder present with at least one (and often multiple) physical symptom. They frequently seek treatment from many doctors, often resulting in extensive lab work, diagnostic procedures, hospitalizations, and/or surgeries.

DIAGNOSIS AND DSM-5 CRITERIA

- One or more somatic symptoms (may be predominantly pain) that are distressing or result in significant disruption.
- Excessive thoughts, feelings, or behaviors related to the somatic symptoms or associated health concerns.
- Lasts at least 6 months.

EPIDEMIOLOGY

- Incidence in females likely greater than males.
- Prevalence in general adult population: 5–7%.
- Risk factors include older age, fewer years of education, lower socioeconomic status, unemployment, and history of traumatic experiences in childhood.

TREATMENT AND PROGNOSIS

- The course tends to be chronic and debilitating. Symptoms may periodically improve and then worsen under stress.
- The patient should have regularly scheduled visits with a single primary care physician, who should minimize unnecessary medical workups and treatments.
- Address psychological issues slowly. Patients will likely resist referral to a mental health professional.

> **KEY FACT**
>
> Somatic symptom disorder patients typically express lots of concern over their condition and chronically perseverate over it. Conversion disorder patients often have an abrupt onset of their neurological symptoms (blindness, etc.) but appear unconcerned.

> **WARDS TIP**
>
> When treating a patient with a somatic symptom disorder, it is important for the psychiatrist to work closely with the patient's primary care physician.

Conversion Disorder (Functional Neurological Symptom Disorder)

Patients with conversion disorder have at least one neurological symptom (sensory or motor) which cannot be fully explained by a neurological condition. Examples include blindness, paralysis, and paresthesia. Patients may be surprisingly calm and unconcerned (*la belle indifference*) when describing their symptoms.

DIAGNOSIS AND DSM-5 CRITERIA

- At least one symptom of altered voluntary motor or sensory function.
- Evidence of incompatibility between the symptom and recognized neurological or medical conditions.
- Not better explained by another medical or mental disorder.
- Causes significant distress or impairment in social or occupational functioning or warrants medical evaluation.
- **Common symptoms:** Paralysis, weakness, blindness, mutism, sensory complaints (paresthesias), seizures, globus sensation (*globus hystericus* or sensation of lump in throat).

> **KEY FACT**
>
> Conversion disorder: patients "convert" psychological distress or conflicts into neurological symptoms.

> **KEY FACT**
>
> Conversion-like presentations in elderly patients have a higher likelihood of representing an underlying neurological deficit.

EPIDEMIOLOGY

- Two to three times more common in women than men.
- Onset at any age, but more often in adolescence or early adulthood.
- High incidence of comorbid neurological, depressive, or anxiety disorders.

TREATMENT AND PROGNOSIS

- The primary treatment is education about the illness. Cognitive-behavioral therapy (CBT), with or without physical therapy, can be used if education alone is not effective.
- While patients often spontaneously recover, the prognosis is poor: symptoms may persist, recur, or worsen in 40–66% of patients.

Illness Anxiety Disorder

DIAGNOSIS AND DSM-5 CRITERIA

- Preoccupation with having or acquiring a serious illness.
- Somatic symptoms are not present, or if present, are mild in intensity.
- High level of anxiety about health.
- Performs excessive health-related behaviors or exhibits maladaptive behaviors.
- Persists for at least **6 months**.
- Not better explained by another mental disorder (such as somatic symptom disorder).

EPIDEMIOLOGY

- Men are affected as often as women.
- Average age of onset 20–30 years.
- Approximately 67% have a coexisting major mental disorder.

TREATMENT

- Regularly scheduled visits with one primary care physician.
- Psychotherapy (primarily CBT).
- Comorbid anxiety and depressive disorders should be treated with selective serotonin reuptake inhibitors (SSRIs) or other appropriate psychotropic medications.

PROGNOSIS

- Chronic but episodic—symptoms may wax and wane periodically.
- Can result in significant disability.
- Up to 60% of patients improve significantly.
- Factors predicting better prognosis include fewer somatic symptoms, shorter duration of illness, and absence of childhood physical punishment.

KEY FACT

Illness anxiety disorder is the only somatic symptom-related disorder that occurs as frequently in men as in women.

Psychological Factors Affecting Other Medical Conditions

A patient with one or more psychological or behavioral factors (e.g., distress, coping styles, maladaptive health behaviors) adversely affecting a medical symptom or condition. Examples include anxiety worsening asthma, denial that acute chest pain needs treatment, and manipulating insulin doses in order to lose weight.

DIAGNOSIS AND DSM-5 CRITERIA

- A medical symptom or condition (other than mental disorder) is present.
- Psychological or behavioral factors adversely affect the medical condition in at least one way, such as influencing the course or treatment, constituting an additional health risk factor, influencing the underlying pathophysiology, precipitating, or exacerbating symptoms or necessitating medical attention.
- Psychological or behavioral factors are not better explained by another mental disorder.

EPIDEMIOLOGY

- Prevalence and gender differences are unclear.
- Can occur across the lifespan.

TREATMENT AND PROGNOSIS

- Treatment includes education and frequent contact with a primary care physician.
- SSRIs and/or psychotherapy (especially CBT) should be used to treat underlying anxiety or depression.

Factitious Disorder

Patients with factitious disorder intentionally falsify medical or psychological signs or symptoms in order to assume the role of a sick patient. They often do this in a way that can cause legitimate danger (central line infections, insulin injections, etc.). The *absence of external rewards* is a prominent feature of this disorder.

DIAGNOSIS AND DSM-5 CRITERIA

- Falsification of physical or psychological signs or symptoms, or induction of injury or disease, associated with identified deception.
- The deceptive behavior is evident even in the absence of obvious external rewards.
- Behavior is not better explained by another mental disorder, such as delusional disorder or another psychotic disorder.
- Individual can present himself/herself, or another individual (as in factitious disorder imposed on another).

KEY FACT

Münchhausen syndrome is another, older name for factitious disorder with predominantly physical complaints. Münchhausen syndrome by proxy is intentionally producing symptoms in someone else who is under one's care (usually one's children).

- **Commonly feigned symptoms:**
  - *Psychiatric*—hallucinations, depression.
  - *Medical*—fever (by heating the thermometer), infection, hypoglycemia, abdominal pain, seizures, and hematuria.

EPIDEMIOLOGY

- May be at least 1% of hospitalized patients.
- More common in women.
- Higher incidence in hospital and health care workers (who have learned how to feign symptoms).
- Associated with personality disorders.
- Many patients have a history of illness and hospitalization, as well as childhood physical or sexual abuse.

TREATMENT AND PROGNOSIS

- Collect collateral information from medical providers and family. Collaborate with primary care physician and treatment team to avoid unnecessary procedures.
- Patients may require confrontation in a nonthreatening manner; however, patients who are confronted may leave against medical advice and seek hospitalization elsewhere.
- Repeated and long-term hospitalizations are common.

Malingering

 A 37-year-old patient claims that he has frequent episodes of "seizures," starts on medications, and joins an epilepsy support group. It becomes known that he is doing this in order to collect social security disability money. *Diagnosis?* **Malingering.** In contrast, in **factitious disorder,** patients look for some kind of unconscious emotional gain by playing the "sick role," such as sympathy from the physician. The fundamental difference between malingering and factitious disorder is in the intention of the patient; in malingering, the motivation is external, whereas in factitious disorder, the motivation is internal.

Malingering involves the intentional reporting of physical or psychological symptoms in order to achieve personal gain. Common external motivations include avoiding the police, receiving room and board, obtaining narcotics, and receiving monetary compensation. Note that malingering is **not** considered a mental illness.

PRESENTATION

- Patients usually present with multiple vague complaints that do not conform to a known medical condition.
- They often have a long medical history with many hospital stays.
- They are generally uncooperative and refuse to accept a good prognosis even after extensive medical evaluation.
- Their symptoms improve once their desired objective is obtained.

EPIDEMIOLOGY

- Not uncommon in hospitalized patients.
- Significantly more common in men than women.

MANAGEMENT

- Work with the patient to manage their underlying distress, if possible.
- Gentle confrontation may be necessary; however, patients who are confronted may leave the hospital AMA and seek treatment elsewhere.

Review of Distinguishing Features

- **Somatic symptom disorders:** Patients *believe* they are ill and do not intentionally produce or feign symptoms.
- **Factitious disorder:** Patients intentionally produce symptoms of a psychological or physical illness because of a desire to assume the *sick role*, not for external rewards.
- **Malingering:** Patients intentionally produce or feign symptoms for *external rewards*.

> **KEY FACT**
>
> Malingering is the *conscious* feigning of symptoms for some secondary gain (e.g., monetary compensation or avoiding incarceration).

CHAPTER 13
IMPULSE CONTROL DISORDERS

Intermittent Explosive Disorder	149
Diagnosis and DSM-5 Criteria	149
Epidemiology/Etiology	149
Treatment	149
Kleptomania	149
Diagnosis and DSM-5 Criteria	149
Epidemiology/Etiology	150
Treatment	150
Pyromania	150
Diagnosis and DSM-5 Criteria	150
Epidemiology/Etiology	150
Treatment	150

Impulse control disorders are characterized by problems in the self-regulation of emotions and behaviors. The behaviors violate the rights of others and/or conflict with societal norms. Impulse control disorders are not caused by another mental disorder, medical condition, or substance use.

Core qualities of the impulse control disorders are as follows:

- Repetitive or compulsive engagement in behavior despite adverse consequences.
- Little control over the negative behavior.
- Anxiety or craving experienced prior to engagement in impulsive behavior.
- Relief or satisfaction during or after completion of the behavior.

Mr. Baker is a 27-year-old married accountant who arrives at the outpatient psychiatry clinic complaining of difficulty in managing his anger. He has no prior psychiatric history, but reports that he has had difficulty controlling his temper since adolescence. He reports that he is easily angered by small occurrences, such as his wife's failing to make coffee or a coworker's forgetting a pen at work. He reacts quickly and in a volatile way, describing it as "going from 0 to 60 before I know it." Mr. Baker feels that he is unable to control his anger; on several occasions he has thrown objects and destroyed property in fits of rage, and has made threatening statements to his wife and coworkers in the past year. Because of these incidents, one coworker has recently threatened to pursue legal action.

Mr. Baker describes these episodes as brief, lasting only 10–15 minutes, and feels embarrassed shortly after the episode has transpired. He is concerned he may lose his job because of his behavior, and he worries about the fate of his relationships. He rarely drinks alcohol, and denies any history of illicit drug use.

What is his most likely diagnosis?

Based on Mr. Baker's history, his most likely diagnosis is intermittent explosive disorder. However, it is important to recognize that impulsivity is a common characteristic of other psychiatric diagnoses, and these must be ruled out prior to diagnosing a patient with this disorder.

What would be your recommended treatment?

Treatment for this disorder usually involves medications to treat impulsive aggression. These include selective serotonin reuptake inhibitors (SSRIs)—fluoxetine being the most studied—and mood stabilizers such as anticonvulsants and lithium. Individual psychotherapy is difficult and has limited efficacy given the nature of the disease and lack of individual control. However, cognitive-behavioral therapy (CBT) has been used in the treatment of anger management. Group therapy and/or family therapy may be useful to create behavior plans to help manage episodes.

What are associated laboratory findings?

In some impulsive individuals, cerebrospinal fluid testing shows low mean 5-hydroxyindoleacetic acid (5-HIAA) concentration. There may also be nonspecific electroencephalographic findings or abnormalities on neuropsychological testing.

Intermittent Explosive Disorder

DIAGNOSIS AND DSM-5 CRITERIA

- Recurrent behavioral outbursts resulting in verbal and/or physical aggression against people or property.

Either:
  - Frequent verbal/physical outbursts (that do not result in physical damage to people, animals, or property) twice weekly for 3 months.

Or:
  - Rare (more than three times per year) outbursts resulting in physical damage to others, animals, or property.
- Outbursts and aggression are grossly out of proportion to the triggering event or stressor.
- Outbursts are not premeditated and not committed to obtain a desired reward.
- Aggressive outbursts cause either marked distress or impairment in occupational/interpersonal functioning, or are associated with financial/legal consequences.
- Aggression is not better explained by another mental disorder, medical condition, or due to the effects of a substance (drug or medication).

EPIDEMIOLOGY/ETIOLOGY

- More common in men than women.
- Onset usually in late childhood or adolescence.
- May be episodic, but course is generally chronic and persistent.
- Genetic, perinatal, environmental, and neurobiological factors may play a role in etiology. Patients may have a history of childhood physical or emotional abuse or head trauma.

KEY FACT

Low levels of serotonin in the CSF have been shown to be associated with impulsiveness and aggression.

TREATMENT

- Treatment involves use of SSRIs, anticonvulsants, or lithium.
- CBT has been shown to be effective and is often used in combination with medications.
- Group therapy and/or family therapy may be useful to create behavior plans to help manage episodes.

Kleptomania

DIAGNOSIS AND DSM-5 CRITERIA

- Failure to resist uncontrollable urges to steal objects that are not needed for personal use or monetary value.
- Increasing internal tension immediately prior to the theft.
- Pleasure or relief is experienced while stealing; however, those with the disorder often report intense guilt and depression.
- Stealing is not committed to express anger/vengeance and does not occur in response to a delusion or hallucination.
- Objects stolen are typically given or thrown away, returned, or hoarded.

> **KEY FACT**
>
> Sixty-five percent of patients with kleptomania suffer from bulimia nervosa.

EPIDEMIOLOGY/ETIOLOGY

- Three times more common in women than men, though rare in the general population.
- Occurs in 4–24% of shoplifters.
- Higher incidence of comorbid mood disorders, eating disorders (especially bulimia nervosa), anxiety disorders, substance use disorders, and personality disorders.
- Higher risk of OCD and substance use disorders in family members.
- Illness usually begins in adolescence and course is episodic.

TREATMENT

Treatment may include CBT (including systematic desensitization and aversive conditioning) and SSRIs. There is also some anecdotal evidence for the use of naltrexone, which blocks reward pathways mediated by endogenous opioids.

Pyromania

DIAGNOSIS AND DSM-5 CRITERIA

- At least two episodes of deliberate fire setting.
- Tension or arousal experienced before the act; pleasure, gratification, or relief experienced when setting fires or witnessing/participating in their aftermath.
- Fascination with, interest in, curiosity about, or attraction to fire and contexts.
- Purpose of fire setting is not for monetary gain, for expression of anger or vengeance, to conceal criminal activity, or as an expression of sociopolitical ideology. It is not in response to a hallucination, delusion, or impaired judgment (intoxication, neurocognitive disorder).
- Fire setting is not better explained by conduct disorder, a manic episode, or antisocial personality disorder.

> **KEY FACT**
>
> Pyromania is the impulse to start fires, typically with feelings of gratification or relief afterward.

EPIDEMIOLOGY/ETIOLOGY

- Rare disorder but much more common in men.
- Most begin to set fires in adolescence or early adulthood.
- High comorbidity with mood disorders, substance use disorders, gambling disorder, and conduct disorder.
- Episodes are episodic and wax and wane in frequency.

TREATMENT

Most don't go into treatment and symptoms will remain chronic. While there is no standard treatment, CBT, SSRIs, mood stabilizers, and antipsychotics have all been used.

NOTES

CHAPTER 14
EATING DISORDERS

Definition	154
Anorexia Nervosa	155
Diagnosis and DSM-5 Criteria	155
Physical findings and medical complications	155
Epidemiology	156
Etiology	156
Differential diagnosis	156
Course and prognosis	156
Treatment	156
Bulimia Nervosa	157
Diagnosis and DSM-5 criteria	157
Physical findings and medical complications	157
Epidemiology	157
Etiology	158
Course and prognosis	158
Treatment	158
Binge-Eating Disorder	158
Diagnosis and DSM-5 criteria	158
Physical findings and medical complications	159
Epidemiology	159
Etiology	159
Course and prognosis	159
Treatment	159

Definition

Eating disorders include anorexia nervosa, bulimia nervosa, and binge-eating disorder. Patients with anorexia or bulimia have a disturbed body image and use extensive measures to avoid gaining weight (vomiting, laxatives, diuretics, enemas, fasting, and excessive exercise). Patients with binge-eating disorder typically binge in response to negative emotions.

> **WARDS TIP**
>
> Suspect an eating disorder? Ask the patient what is the most/least he/she has weighed, his/her ideal body weight, if he/she counts calories/fat/carbs/protein, how much he/she exercises, if he/she binges and purges, and if he/she has food rituals (e.g., drinking water between bites).

 Ms. Williams is a 17-year-old Caucasian woman without prior psychiatric history who is brought to the emergency room by ambulance after her parents called 911 when they found her having a seizure in their living room. She was admitted to the medical intensive care unit in status epilepticus and was quickly stabilized with intramuscular lorazepam and fosphenytoin loading. Her height is 5 feet 6 inches, she is of medium build, and her weight is 101 pounds (BMI 16.3 kg/m^2). She has no significant medical history, and this is her first seizure. Laboratory workup shows an electrolyte imbalance as the most likely cause for her seizures. Although initially reluctant, she admits to self-induced vomiting several times this week. She reports that although she normally restricts her daily caloric intake to 500 calories, she regularly induces vomiting if her weight is above 100 pounds. Her last menstrual cycle was 1 year ago. Psychiatric consultation is requested in order to confirm her diagnosis.

As the psychiatrist on call, you evaluate Ms. Williams and find that she appears underweight and younger than her stated age. She is in mild distress, has a nasogastric tube in place, and exhibits poor eye contact. She reports feeling "sad" and admits to experiencing constant preoccupation about her physical appearance, stating "I'm fat. I hate my body." She also reports insomnia, low energy levels, and a history of self-harm behavior by cutting her forearms. She reports that she is careful in hiding her symptoms from her parents, whom she describes as strict disciplinarians. She also expresses concerns that she will disappoint them.

Ms. Williams's parents describe her as a perfectionist. They say that she is involved in multiple school activities, takes advanced placement classes, and has been recently concerned about being accepted to her college of choice. They report that she has maintained a 4.0 grade point average in high school, and they expect her to become a doctor. Her parents have noticed that she is underweight and rarely see her eat, but have attributed this to stress from her many academic pursuits. Ms. Williams's mother receives treatment for obsessive-compulsive disorder.

What is Ms. Williams's most likely diagnosis?

The most likely diagnosis is anorexia nervosa—binge-eating/purging type. As described above, she refuses to weigh more than 100 pounds, which is significantly below the minimal normal weight for her height. Despite being underweight, she expresses intense fear of gaining weight and has a disturbance in the way her body shape is experienced. In addition, she has engaged in binge-eating/purging behavior regularly. You should also explore for comorbid depression, anxiety, and a personality disorder. Remember that malnutrition in itself can lead to some of the symptoms experienced in depression, and that many patients show an improvement in their mood when nutrition is replenished.

What are some of the medical complications associated with this condition?

Patients with anorexia nervosa can present with bradycardia, orthostatic hypotension, arrhythmias, QTc prolongation, and ST-T wave changes on electrocardiogram, as well as anemia and leukopenia. They may also experience cognitive impairment, evidence of enlarged ventricles and/or decrease in gray and white matter on brain imaging, and peripheral neuropathy. Lanugo and muscle wasting sometimes become evident. Amenorrhea and loss of libido are commonly reported. In patients who regularly engage in self-induced vomiting, parotid enlargement, increased amylase levels, and electrolyte imbalances (e.g., hypokalemia) not uncommonly occur as a result.

Anorexia Nervosa

Patients with anorexia nervosa are preoccupied with their weight, their body image, and being thin. It is often associated with obsessive-compulsive personality traits. There are two main subtypes:

- **Restricting type:** Has not regularly engaged in binge-eating or purging behavior; weight loss is achieved through diet, fasting, and/or excessive exercise.
- **Binge-eating/purging type:** Eating binges followed by self-induced vomiting, and/or using laxatives, enemas, or diuretics. Some individuals purge after eating small amounts of food without binging.

KEY FACT

Both anorexia and bulimia are characterized by a desire for thinness. Both may binge and purge. Anorexia nervosa involves low body weight and restriction of calorie intake, and this distinguishes it from bulimia.

DIAGNOSIS AND DSM-5 CRITERIA

- Restriction of energy intake relative to requirements, leading to significant low body weight—defined as less than minimally normal or expected.
- Intense fear of gaining weight or becoming fat, or persistent behaviors that prevent weight gain.
- Disturbed body image, undue influence of weight or shape on self-evaluation, or denial of the seriousness of the current low body weight.

KEY FACT

Classic example of anorexia nervosa: An extremely thin teenage girl with amenorrhea, whose mother says she eats very little, does aerobics for 2 hours a day, and *ritualistically* performs 400 sit-ups every day (500 if she has "overeaten").

PHYSICAL FINDINGS AND MEDICAL COMPLICATIONS

- The medical complications of eating disorders are related to weight loss and purging (e.g., vomiting and laxative abuse).
- Physical manifestations: Amenorrhea, cold intolerance/hypothermia, hypotension (especially orthostasis), bradycardia, arrhythmia, acute coronary syndrome, cardiomyopathy, mitral valve prolapse, constipation, lanugo (fine, soft body hair typically found in newborns), alopecia, edema, dehydration, peripheral neuropathy, seizures, hypothyroidism, osteopenia, osteoporosis.
- Laboratory/imaging abnormalities: Hyponatremia, hypochloremic hypokalemic alkalosis (if vomiting), arrhythmia (especially QTc prolongation), hypercholesterolemia, transaminitis, leukopenia, anemia (normocytic

normochromic), elevated blood urea nitrogen (BUN), increased growth hormone (GH), increased cortisol, reduced gonadotropins (luteinizing hormone [LH], follicle-stimulating hormone [FSH]), reduced sex steroid hormones (estrogen, testosterone), hypothyroidism, hypoglycemia, osteopenia.

EPIDEMIOLOGY

- Ten to one female to male ratio. Twelve-month prevalence among young females is 0.4%.
- Bimodal age of onset (age 13–14: hormonal influences; age 17–18: environmental influences). More common in industrialized countries where food is abundant and a thin body ideal is held.
- Common in sports that involve thinness, revealing attire, subjective judging, and weight classes (e.g., running, ballet, wrestling, diving, cheerleading, figure skating).

ETIOLOGY

- Multifactorial.
- Genetics: Higher concordance in monozygotic than dizygotic twin studies.
- Psychodynamic theories: Difficulty with separation and autonomy (e.g., parental enmeshment), and struggle to gain control.
- Social theories: Exaggeration of social values (achievement, control, and perfectionism), idealization of thin body and prepubescent appearance in Western world, increased prevalence of dieting at earlier ages.

DIFFERENTIAL DIAGNOSIS

- Medical conditions: Endocrine disorders (e.g., hypothalamic disease, diabetes mellitus, hyperthyroidism), gastrointestinal illnesses (e.g., malabsorption, inflammatory bowel disease), genetic disorders (e.g., Turner syndrome, Gaucher disease), cancer, AIDS.
- Psychiatric disorders: Major depression, bulimia, or other mental disorders (such as somatic symptom disorder or schizophrenia).

COURSE AND PROGNOSIS

- Chronic and relapsing illness. Variable course—may completely recover, have fluctuating symptoms with relapses, or progressively deteriorate. Most remit within 5 years.
- Mortality rate is cumulative and approximately 5% per decade due to starvation, **suicide,** or cardiac failure. Rates of suicide are approximately 12 per 100,000 per year.

TREATMENT

- Food is the best medicine.
- Patients may be treated as outpatients unless they are dangerously below ideal body weight (>20–25% below) or if there are serious medical or

KEY FACT

Anorexia versus Major Depressive Disorder: Appetite
Anorexia nervosa: Patients have a *good appetite* but starve themselves due to distorted body image. They are often quite preoccupied with food (e.g., preparing it for others) but do not eat it themselves.
Major depressive disorder: Patients usually have *poor appetite,* which leads to weight loss. These patients have no or decreased interest in food.

KEY FACT

Refeeding syndrome refers to electrolyte and fluid shifts that occur when severely malnourished patients are refed too quickly. Look for fluid retention and decreased levels of phosphorus, magnesium, and calcium. Complications include arrhythmias, respiratory failure, delirium, and seizures. Replace electrolytes and slow the feedings.

WARDS TIP

When a patient with anorexia learns that weight gain is a common side effect, he/she may refuse medication.

psychiatric complications, in which case they should be hospitalized for supervised refeeding.
- Treatment involves cognitive-behavioral therapy, family therapy (e.g., Maudsley approach—the gold standard for treatment of anorexia nervosa in teenagers), and supervised weight-gain programs.
- Selective serotonin reuptake inhibitors (SSRIs) have not been effective in the treatment of anorexia nervosa but may be used for comorbid anxiety or depression.
- Little evidence that second-generation antipsychotics can treat preoccupation with weight and food, or independently promote weight gain. Olanzapine has the most evidence in this regard.
- There is some consensus that a premeal anxiolytic (such as alprazolam) can help encourage eating by decreasing anticipatory anxiety.

WARDS TIP

Unlike patients with anorexia nervosa, bulimic patients usually maintain a normal weight (or are overweight) and their symptoms are more ego-dystonic (distressing); they are therefore more likely to seek help.

Bulimia Nervosa

Bulimia nervosa involves binge eating combined with behaviors intended to counteract weight gain, such as vomiting; use of laxatives, enemas, or diuretics; fasting; or excessive exercise. Patients are embarrassed by their binge eating and are overly concerned with body weight. However, unlike patients with anorexia, they usually maintain a normal weight (and may be overweight).

DIAGNOSIS AND DSM-5 CRITERIA

- Recurrent episodes of binge eating.
- Recurrent, inappropriate attempts to compensate for overeating and prevent weight gain (such as laxative abuse, vomiting, diuretics, fasting, or excessive exercise).
- The binge eating and compensatory behaviors occur at least once a week for 3 months.
- Perception of self-worth is excessively influenced by body weight and shape.
- Does not occur exclusively during an episode of anorexia nervosa.

PHYSICAL FINDINGS AND MEDICAL COMPLICATIONS

- Patients with anorexia and bulimia may have similar medical complications related to weight loss and vomiting.
- Physical manifestations: Salivary gland enlargement (sialadenosis), dental erosion/caries, callouses/abrasions on dorsum of hand ("Russell's sign" from self-induced vomiting), petechiae, peripheral edema, aspiration.
- Laboratory/imaging abnormalities: Hypochloremic hypokalemic alkalosis, metabolic acidosis (laxative abuse), elevated bicarbonate (compensation), hypernatremia, increased BUN, increased amylase, altered thyroid hormone, cortisol homeostasis, esophagitis.

EPIDEMIOLOGY

- Twelve-month prevalence in young females is 1–1.5%.
- Significantly more common in women than men (10:1 ratio).

KEY FACT

Binge eating is defined by excessive food intake within a 2-hour period accompanied by a sense of lack of control.

KEY FACT

Anorexia nervosa and bulimia nervosa are risk factors for developing cardiac arrhythmias due to electrolyte disturbances such as hypokalemia.

KEY FACT

Compared to patients with bulimia nervosa, cortisol is often increase in patients with anorexia nervosa.

- Onset is in late adolescence or early adulthood.
- More common in developed countries.
- High incidence of comorbid mood disorders, anxiety disorders, impulse control disorders, substance use, prior physical/sexual abuse, and increased prevalence of borderline personality disorder.

ETIOLOGY

- Multifactorial, with similar factors as for anorexia (e.g., genetic and social theories).
- Childhood obesity and early pubertal maturation increase risk for bulimia nervosa.
- Psychodynamic theories: Masochistic displays of control and displaced anger over one's body.

COURSE AND PROGNOSIS

- Chronic and relapsing illness.
- Better prognosis than anorexia nervosa.
- Symptoms are usually exacerbated by stressful conditions.
- One-half recover fully with treatment; one-half have chronic course with fluctuating symptoms.
- Crude mortality rate is 2% per decade.
- Elevated suicide risk compared to the general population.

TREATMENT

- Antidepressants plus therapy are more efficacious for treating bulimia nervosa than either treatment alone.
- SSRIs are first-line medication.
- Fluoxetine is the only Food and Drug Administration (FDA)-approved medication for bulimia (60–80 mg/day).
- Nutritional counseling and education.
- Therapy includes cognitive-behavioral therapy, interpersonal psychotherapy, group therapy, and family therapy. Cognitive behavioral therapy has demonstrated more efficacy than the other therapies.
- Avoid bupropion due to its potential side effect to lower seizure threshold.

KEY FACT

Classic example of bulimia nervosa: A 20-year-old college student is referred by her dentist because of multiple dental caries. She is normal weight for her height but feels that "she needs to lose 15 pounds." She reluctantly admits to eating large quantities of food in a short period of time and then inducing vomiting.

KEY FACT

Fluoxetine is an effective medication for bulimia.

WARDS TIP

In patients with bulimia, make sure to check that they aren't on medications that could further lower their seizure threshold, such as the antidepressant Wellbutrin (bupropion).

Binge-Eating Disorder

Patients with binge-eating disorder suffer emotional distress over their binge eating, but they do not try to control their weight by purging or restricting calories, as do individuals with anorexia or bulimia. Unlike in anorexia and bulimia, patients with binge-eating disorder are not as fixated on their body shape and weight.

DIAGNOSIS AND DSM-5 CRITERIA

- Recurrent episodes of binge eating (eating an excessive amount of food in a 2-hour period associated with a lack of control), with at least three of

the following: eating very rapidly, eating until uncomfortably full, eating large amounts when not hungry, eating alone due to embarrassment, and feeling disgusted/depressed/guilty after eating.
- Severe distress over binge eating.
- Binge eating occurs at least once a week for 3 months.
- Binge eating is not associated with compensatory behaviors (such as vomiting and laxative use), and doesn't occur exclusively during the course of anorexia or bulimia.

PHYSICAL FINDINGS AND MEDICAL COMPLICATIONS

Patients are typically obese and suffer from medical problems related to obesity including metabolic syndrome, type 2 diabetes, and cardiovascular disease.

EPIDEMIOLOGY

- Twelve-month prevalence is 1.6% for females and 0.8% for males.
- Equal prevalence in females across ethnicities.
- Increased prevalence among individuals seeking weight-loss treatment compared to the general population.

ETIOLOGY

Runs in families, reflecting likely genetic influences.

COURSE AND PROGNOSIS

- Typically begins in adolescence or young adulthood.
- Appears to be relatively persistent, though remission rates are higher than for other eating disorders.
- Most obese individuals do not binge eat; those who do have more functional impairment, lower quality of life, and more subjective distress than weight matched controls.
- Higher rates of psychiatric comorbidities than in obese individuals without binge-eating disorder.

TREATMENT

- Treatment involves individual (cognitive-behavioral or interpersonal) psychotherapy with a strict diet and exercise program coordinated by a registered dietician. Comorbid mood disorders or anxiety disorders should be treated as necessary.
- **SSRIs are first-line treatment due to their efficacy and tolerability.**
- Although not frequently used due to significant side effects and limited long-term efficacy, pharmacotherapy may be used adjunctively to directly promote weight loss:
  - Lisdexamfetamine (Vyvanse)—stimulant that suppresses appetite and is FDA-approved for the treatment of binge-eating disorder.
  - Topiramate and zonisimide—antiepileptics associated with weight loss.
  - Orlistat (Xenical)—inhibits pancreatic lipase, thus decreasing amount of fat absorbed from the gastrointestinal tract.

CHAPTER 14 EATING DISORDERS

NOTES

CHAPTER 15

SLEEP-WAKE DISORDERS

Normal Sleep-Wake Cycle	162
Sleep Disorders	162
Dyssomnias	162
Insomnia Disorder	163
Hypersomnolence Disorder	164
Obstructive Sleep Apnea Hypopnea	165
Central Sleep Apnea	165
Sleep-Related Hypoventilation	166
Narcolepsy	167
Circadian Rhythm Sleep-Wake Disorders	168
Parasomnias	168
Non-REM Sleep Arousal Disorders	169
Sleepwalking	169
Sleep Terrors	170
Nightmare Disorder	170
REM Sleep Behavior Disorder	171
Restless Legs Syndrome	172
Substance/Medication-Induced Sleep Disorder	172

Sleep disorders affect as many as 40% of the U.S. adult population. Current data demonstrate a high rate of comorbidity between sleep disorders and various psychiatric illnesses. Disturbances in sleep can potentiate and/or exacerbate psychological distress and other mental illnesses.

Normal Sleep-Wake Cycle

- Normal sleep-wake cycle is defined in terms of characteristic changes in several physiological parameters, including brain wave activity, eye movements, and motor activity.
- The two stages of normal sleep are rapid eye movement (REM) sleep and non-rapid eye movement (NREM) sleep.
- About every 90 minutes, NREM sleep alternates with REM sleep.
- NREM induces transition from the waking state to deep sleep.
- Progression through NREM sleep results in slower brain wave patterns and higher arousal thresholds.
- In REM sleep, brain wave patterns resemble the electroencephalogram (EEG) of an aroused person.
- Awakening from REM sleep is associated with vivid dream recall.

FIGURE 15-1. **The sleep cycle.** © 2008 LLS. Adapted, with permission of the publisher, Les Laboratoires Servier, from Figure 1 in Nutt D, Wilson S, Paterson L. Sleep disorders as core symptoms of depression. Dialogues Clin Neurosci. 2008; 10(3): 329-336.

Sleep Disorders

- Classified as either:
    - **Dyssomnias:** Insufficient, excessive, or altered timing of sleep.
    - **Parasomnias:** Unusual sleep-related behaviors.
- When taking a sleep history, ask about:
    - **A**ctivities prior to bedtime that may interfere with restful sleep.
    - **B**ed partner history.
    - **C**onsequence on waking function; quality of life.
    - **D**rug regimen, medications.
    - **E**xacerbating or relieving factors.
    - **F**requency and duration.
    - **G**enetic factors or family history.
    - **H**abits (alcohol consumption, use of caffeine, nicotine, illicit substances, and hypnotics).

Dyssomnias

Dyssomnias are disorders that make it difficult to fall or remain asleep (insomnias), or of excessive daytime sleeping (hypersomnias).

INSOMNIA DISORDER

- Refers to a number of symptoms that interfere with duration and/or quality of sleep despite adequate opportunity for sleep. Symptoms may include:
  - Difficulty initiating sleep (*initial or sleep-onset insomnia*).
  - Frequent nocturnal awakenings (*middle or sleep-maintenance insomnia*).
  - Early morning awakenings (*late or sleep-offset insomnia*).
  - Waking up feeling fatigued and unrefreshed (*nonrestorative sleep*).
- **Acute insomnia** (less than 3 months) is generally associated with stress or changes in sleep schedule and usually resolves spontaneously.
- **Chronic insomnia** lasts more than or equal to 3 months to years and is associated with reduced quality of life and increased risk of psychiatric illness.
- **Diagnosis is often assisted by use of subjective sleep tracking measures such as the Consensus Sleep Diary.**

DSM-5 Criteria

- Difficulty initiating/maintaining sleep or early-morning awakening with inability to return to sleep.
- Occurs at least 3 days a week for at least 3 months.
- Causes clinically significant distress or impairment in functioning.
- Occurs despite adequate opportunity to sleep.
- Does not occur exclusively during the course of another sleep-wake disorder.
- Not due to the physiologic effects of a substance or medication.
- Coexisting mental and medical disorders do not adequately explain the insomnia.

Epidemiology

Prevalence: 6–10% (the most prevalent of all sleep-wake disorders).

Etiology

- Subclinical mood and/or anxiety disorders.
- Preoccupation with a perceived inability to sleep.
- Bedtime behavior not conducive to adequate sleep (**poor sleep hygiene**).
- Idiopathic.

Treatment

- Sleep hygiene measures.
- Cognitive-behavioral therapy (CBT).
- Chronotherapy (bright light therapy) has evidence supporting its use in treating insomnia by entraining the circadian rhythm.
- Pharmacotherapy:
  - Benzodiazepines:
    - Reduce sleep latency and nocturnal awakening.
    - As effective as CBT during short periods of treatment (4–8 weeks); insufficient evidence to support long-term efficacy.
    - Side effects include development of tolerance, addiction, daytime sleepiness, and rebound insomnia.
    - In the elderly, falls, confusion, and dizziness are of particular concern.

> **KEY FACT**
>
> REM sleep is characterized by increase in blood pressure, heart rate, and respiratory rate.

> **KEY FACT**
>
> CBT is considered first-line therapy for chronic insomnia.

> **KEY FACT**
>
> Insomnia is the most common reason patients are put on long-term benzodiazepines.

- Non-benzodiazepines:
  - Include melatonin, zolpidem (Ambien), eszopiclone (Lunesta), zaleplon (Sonata), and suvorexant (Belsomra).
  - Effective for short-term treatment.
  - Associated with low incidence of daytime sleepiness and orthostatic hypotension.
  - In the elderly, zolpidem causes increased risk of falls and may induce cognitive impairment.
  - Doses of zolpidem more than 10 mg can cause increase in cognitive impairment in women.
- Antidepressants:
  - Trazodone, amitriptyline, and doxepin (off-label use).
  - Mirtazapine (in low doses) is often used to promote sleep in patients with coexisting depressive disorders.
  - Side effects include sedation, dizziness, and psychomotor impairment.
  - Trazodone is the most prescribed sedating antidepressant for patients with chronic insomnia and depressive symptoms.

KEY FACT

Breathing-related disorders are the most common of the hypersomnias and include obstructive sleep apnea and central sleep apnea.

HYPERSOMNOLENCE DISORDER

- Refers to symptoms of excessive quantity of sleep, reduced quality of wakefulness, and sleep inertia/*sleep drunkenness* (i.e., impaired performance and reduced alertness after awakening).
- Complain of nonrestorative sleep, automatic behaviors (routine behavior performed with little to no recall), and difficulty awakening in the morning.

DSM-5 Criteria

- Excessive sleepiness despite at least 7 hours of sleep, with at least one of the following: recurrent periods of sleep within the same day; prolonged, nonrestorative sleep more than 9 hours; difficulty being fully awake after awakening.
- Occurs at least three times per week for at least 3 months.
- Causes clinically significant distress or impairment in functioning.
- Does not occur exclusively during the course of another sleep-wake disorder.
- Not due to the physiologic effects of a substance or medication.
- Coexisting mental and medical disorders do not adequately explain the hypersomnolence.

Epidemiology

- Prevalence: 5–10% of individuals presenting to sleep disorders clinics.
- Equal frequency in men and women.

Etiology

- Viral infections (e.g., HIV pneumonia, infectious mononucleosis, Guillain–Barré).
- Head trauma.
- Genetic—may have autosomal dominant mode of inheritance in some individuals.

Course

- Progressive onset, beginning between ages 15 and 25.
- Persistent course unless treated.

Treatment
- Life-long therapy with modafinil or stimulants such as methylphenidate; amphetamine-like antidepressants such as atomoxetine are second-line therapy.
- Pitolisant (Wakix) and sodium oxybate (Xyrem) have shown benefit as well.
- Scheduled napping.

OBSTRUCTIVE SLEEP APNEA HYPOPNEA

Chronic breathing-related disorder characterized by repetitive collapse of the upper airway during sleep and evidence by polysomnography of multiple episodes of apnea or hypopnea per hour of sleep.

> A 40-year-old businessman states that over the past 2 years he has had trouble staying awake for more than 2 hours before eventually falling asleep. He then has a hard time sleeping through the night. As a result, his performance at work is suffering. *Diagnosis?* Many possible diagnoses, but you must always consider obstructive sleep apnea in addition to insomnia disorder, narcolepsy, etc.

Features
- Excessive daytime sleepiness.
- Apneic episodes characterized by cessation of breathing or hypopneic episodes of reduced airflow (more than 15 per hour).
- Sleep fragmentation.
- Snoring.
- Frequent awakenings due to gasping or choking.
- Nonrefreshing sleep or fatigue.
- Morning headaches.
- Hypertension.

Risk Factors
Obesity, increased neck circumference, airway narrowing.

Prevalence
- Most common in middle-aged men and women.
- Male to female ratio ranges from 2:1 to 4:1.
- Children: 1–2%; middle-aged adults: 2–15%; older adults: >20%.

Treatment
- Positive airway pressure: continuous (CPAP) and in some cases bilevel (BiPAP).
- Behavioral strategies such as weight loss and exercise.
- Surgery, including tonsillectomy and selective upper airway stimulation implants.

CENTRAL SLEEP APNEA

Evidenced by five or more central apneas per hour of sleep. It can be idiopathic, with Cheyne–Stokes breathing (pattern of periodic crescendo–decrescendo variation in tidal volume due to heart failure, stroke, or renal failure), or due to opioid use. It is associated with insomnia and daytime sleepiness.

Prevalence

- Idiopathic subtype rare.
- Cheyne–Stokes subtype increased in patients with decreased ejection fraction and acute stroke.
- Thirty percent of chronic opioid users have central sleep apnea.
- Higher frequency in men than women.

Course

- Tied to comorbid medical conditions, although may be transient.
- May be chronic in opioid users.

Treatment

- Treat the underlying condition.
- CPAP/BiPAP.
- Supplemental O_2.
- Medications (e.g., acetazolamide [Diamox], theophylline, sedative-hypnotics).

SLEEP-RELATED HYPOVENTILATION

Polysomnography demonstrates decreased respiration and elevated CO_2 levels. Individuals report frequent arousals, morning headaches, insomnia, and excessive daytime sleepiness. Frequently comorbid with medical or neurologic disorders, medication use, or substance use disorder. Over time it can result in pulmonary hypertension, cor pulmonale, cardiac arrhythmias, polycythemia, neurocognitive dysfunction, and eventually respiratory failure due to severe blood gas abnormalities.

Prevalence

Very uncommon.

Course

Slowly progressive.

Treatment

- Treat the underlying condition.
- CPAP/BiPAP.
- Medications to stimulate/promote breathing (e.g., bronchodilators, theophylline).

Mr. Richards is a 22-year-old college student with a history of persistent depressive disorder (dysthymic disorder) who arrives at the outpatient psychiatry clinic complaining of daytime sleepiness. He reports that during the past 2 years, he has fallen asleep while in social situations and during his college classes. He often takes naps during class, in movie theaters, and sometimes in the middle of conversations with his girlfriend. His naps typically last for 5–10 minutes and he awakens feeling better. However, within the next 2–3 hours he feels sleepy again. His colleagues joke about his tendency to sleep everywhere, and he feels embarrassed by this.

Mr. Richards also complains of "weird" experiences while sleeping. He reports that he sometimes sees bright colors and hears loud sounds that feel real to him. He says that when this occurs it is difficult to distinguish if he is dreaming or is awake. He feels frightened by these experiences because he is unable to move when they happen. However, after a few minutes he reports that these feelings resolve, and he is able to move and is fully awake.

In performing a thorough history, you learn that he has had episodes during which he has experienced weakness and has dropped objects from his hands while laughing or becoming angry. Last week, his legs buckled and he fell to the ground after his friends startled him at a surprise birthday party. He denies ever losing consciousness during these episodes, and there have been no reports of witnessed convulsions.

What is this patient's diagnosis?

This patient's symptoms are consistent with a diagnosis of narcolepsy. The classic narcolepsy tetrad (all four present in less than 25% of patients) consists of excessive daytime sleepiness or "sleep attacks," REM-related sleep phenomena including inability to move during the transition from sleep to wakefulness, hypnagogic or hypnopompic hallucinations, and a sudden loss of muscle tone evoked by strong emotion without loss of consciousness (cataplexy). Cataplexy may be mild, affecting only the voice, face, or arms, or generalized, causing patients to fall to the ground, and it occurs in 70% of those diagnosed with narcolepsy.

What are Mr. Richards's treatment options?

In the treatment of narcolepsy, it is important for patients to schedule daytime naps and to maintain a regular sleep schedule at night. They should get at least 8 hours of sleep and keep consistent times for sleeping and awakening. Pharmacological treatments may include the use of stimulants (methylphenidate) and antidepressants. The stimulant modafinil and sodium oxybate (non-stimulant) are also effective in the treatment of narcolepsy. Sodium oxybate (Xyrem) is particularly effective in the treatment of cataplexy.

NARCOLEPSY

Narcolepsy is characterized by excessive daytime sleepiness and falling asleep at inappropriate times.

DSM-5 Criteria

- Recurrent episodes of need to sleep, lapsing into sleep, or napping during the day, occurring at least three times per week for at least 3 months associated with at least one of the following:
    - Cataplexy (brief episodes of sudden bilateral loss of muscle tone, most often associated with intense emotion).
    - Hypocretin deficiency in the CSF.
    - Reduced REM sleep latency on polysomnography.
- Hallucinations and/or sleep paralysis at the beginning or end of sleep episodes are common (but not necessary for diagnosis in the *DSM-5*).

KEY FACT

Hyp**na**gogic hallucination: when *going to* sleep.
Hypono**pom**pic hallucination: when transitioning *from* sleep.

KEY FACT

Don't confuse narcoleptic cataplexy with catatonic catalepsy (unprovoked muscular rigidity).

Epidemiology/Prevalence
- Narcolepsy with cataplexy occurs in 0.02–0.04% worldwide.
- Slightly more common in males than females.

Pathophysiology
- Linked to a loss of hypothalamic neurons that produce hypocretin.
- May have autoimmune component.

Treatment
- Sleep hygiene.
- Scheduled daytime naps.
- Avoidance of shift work.
- For excessive daytime sleepiness:
    - Amphetamines (D-amphetamine, methamphetamine).
    - Non-amphetamines such as methylphenidate, modafinil, sodium oxybate, and pitolisant (a novel histamine H3 receptor inverse agonist that is effective for both daytime sleepiness and cataplexy).
- For cataplexy:
    - Sodium oxybate (drug of choice).
    - Tricyclic antidepressants (TCAs): Imipramine, desipramine, and clomipramine.
    - **REM suppression drugs** such as selective serotonin reuptake inhibitor (SSRI)/serotonin-norepinephrine reuptake inhibitor (SNRI): Fluoxetine, duloxetine, atomoxetine, venlafaxine.
- **Sedative hypnotics are given in some cases to correct disturbed nighttime sleep.**

KEY FACT

The suprachiasmic nucleus (SCN) in the hypothalamus coordinates 24-hour or circadian rhythmicity.

CIRCADIAN RHYTHM SLEEP-WAKE DISORDERS

Circadian rhythm sleep-wake disorders are recurrent patterns of sleep disruption due to an alteration of the circadian system or misalignment between the endogenous circadian rhythm and sleep-wake schedule required by an individual's environment or schedule. Subtypes include delayed sleep phase, advanced sleep phase, irregular sleep-wake, non-24-hour sleep-wake, and shift work (see Table 15-1).

Symptoms
- Excessive daytime sleepiness.
- Insomnia.
- Sleep inertia.
- Headaches.
- Difficulty concentrating.
- Increased reaction times and frequent performance errors.
- Irritability.
- Waking up at inappropriate times.

Parasomnias

- Abnormal behaviors, experiences, or physiological events that occur during sleep or sleep-wake transitions.
- Symptoms may include abnormal movements, emotions, dreams, and autonomic activity.
- Isolated episodes common in childhood and adolescence.
- Include non-REM sleep arousal disorders, nightmare disorder, REM sleep behavior disorder, restless leg syndrome.

TABLE 15-1. Circadian Rhythm Sleep Wake Disorders

Disorders	Definitions	Risk Factors	Treatments
Delayed sleep phase disorder (DPSD)	Chronic or recurrent delay in sleep onset and awakening times with preserved quality and duration of sleep	▪ Puberty (secondary to temporal changes in melatonin secretion) ▪ Caffeine and nicotine use ▪ Irregular sleep schedules	▪ Timed bright light phototherapy during early morning ▪ Administration of melatonin in the evening ▪ Chronotherapy (delaying bedtime by a few hours each night)
Advanced sleep phase disorder	Normal duration and quality of sleep with sleep onset and awakening times earlier than desired	Older age	▪ Timed bright light phototherapy prior to bedtime ▪ Early morning melatonin not recommended (may cause daytime sedation)
Shift-work disorder (SWD)	Sleep deprivation and misalignment of the circadian rhythm secondary to nontraditional work hours	▪ Night shift work ▪ Rotating shifts ▪ Shifts >16 hours ▪ Being a medical/psychiatry resident	▪ Avoid risk factors ▪ Bright light phototherapy to facilitate rapid adaptation to night shift ▪ Modafinil may be helpful for patients with severe SWD
Jet lag disorder	Sleep disturbances (insomnia, hypersomnia) associated with travel across multiple time zones	Recent sleep deprivation	▪ Disorder is usually self-limiting. ▪ Sleep disturbances generally resolve 2–3 days after travel.

NON-REM SLEEP AROUSAL DISORDERS

Repeated episodes of incomplete arousals that are brief and usually occur during the first one-third of the sleep episode. Include sleepwalking and sleep terrors.

SLEEPWALKING

Features
- Repeated episodes of simple to complex behaviors that occur during slow-wave sleep.
- Behaviors may include sitting up in bed, walking around, eating, and in some cases "escaping" outdoors.
- Eyes are usually open with a blank stare and "glassy look."
- Difficulty arousing the sleepwalker during an episode.
- Dreams aren't remembered and there is amnesia for the episode.
- Episodes usually end with patients returning to bed or awakening (briefly) confused and disoriented.
- Rare cases associated with violent behavior.

Epidemiology
- One to seven percent of adults have sleepwalking episodes (not disorder).
- Ten to thirty percent of children have at least one episode and 2–3% sleepwalk often.

Risk Factors
- Sleep deprivation.
- Irregular sleep schedules.

- Stress.
- Fatigue.
- Obstructive sleep apnea.
- Nocturnal seizures.
- Fever.
- Medications, including sedatives/hypnotics, lithium, and anticholinergics.
- Family history.

Etiology

- Unknown.
- Family history in 80% of cases.
- Usually not associated with any significant underlying psychiatric or psychological problems.

Treatment

- Most cases do not need to be treated.
- Patients may benefit from education, reassurance, addressing precipitating factors, ensuring a safe environment, and proper sleep hygiene.
- Refractory cases may respond to low-dose benzodiazepine (e.g., clonazepam).

SLEEP TERRORS

Features

- Recurrent episodes of sudden terror arousals, usually beginning with screaming or crying, that occur during slow-wave sleep.
- Signs of autonomic arousal, including tachycardia, tachypnea, diaphoresis, and mydriasis.
- Difficulty arousing during an episode.
- After episode, patients usually return to sleep without awakening.
- Dreams aren't remembered and there is amnesia for the episode.
- In rare cases, awakening elicits aggressive behavior.

Epidemiology

- Approximately 2% of adults and 20% of young children have sleep terrors (not disorder).
- Tenfold increase in first-degree biological relatives of affected patients.
- High comorbidity with sleepwalking.

Risk Factors

- Same as for sleepwalking.
- Other sleep disorder such as sleep apnea.

Treatment

- Reassurance that the condition is benign and self-limited.
- Same as for sleepwalking.

NIGHTMARE DISORDER

Features

- Recurrent frightening dreams that occur during the second half of the sleep episode.
- Terminate in awakening with vivid recall.

- No confusion or disorientation upon awakening.
- Causes clinically significant distress or impairment in functioning.

Epidemiology

- Frequent nightmares in 1–2% of adults, higher prevalence in women.
- Peak prevalence in late adolescence or early adulthood.
- Nightmares are seen in at least 50–70% of posttraumatic stress disorder (PTSD) cases.

Treatment

- Not always needed. Reassurance may help in many cases.
- **Desensitization/Imagery rehearsal therapy** (IRT) involves the use of mental imagery to modify the outcome of a recurrent nightmare, writing down the improved outcome, and then mentally rehearsing it in a relaxed state.
- **Medications are rarely indicated**. Prazosin and antidepressants are often used to treat nightmares related to PTSD.

WARDS TIP

Imagery rehearsal therapy (IRT) has been successful in treating recurrent nightmares in patients with PTSD.

REM SLEEP BEHAVIOR DISORDER

Features

- Repeated arousals during sleep associated with vocalization or complex motor behavior (dream enacting behaviors) occurring during REM, more often in the second half of the sleep episode.
- Characterized by lack of muscle atonia during REM sleep.
- No confusion or disorientation upon awakening.
- Dream-enacting behaviors include:
    - Sleep talking.
    - Yelling.
    - Limb jerking.
    - Walking and/or running.
    - Punching and/or other violent behaviors.
- Presenting complaint is often violent behaviors during sleep resulting in injury to the patient and/or to the bed partner.

Epidemiology

- Prevalence in general population is approximately 0.5%, likely higher in people with psychiatric disorders.
- Occurs mostly in males.

Risk Factors

- Older age, generally more than 50 years.
- Psychiatric medications such as TCAs, SSRIs, SNRIs, and β-blockers.
- Narcolepsy.
- Highly associated with underlying neurodegenerative disorders, especially Parkinson's, multiple system atrophy, and neurocognitive disorder with Lewy bodies.

Treatment

- Discontinuation of likely causative medications if possible.
- Clonazepam is efficacious in most patients.
- Melatonin may also be helpful.
- Ensure environmental safety such as removing potentially dangerous objects from the bedroom and sleeping on the ground until behaviors can be managed effectively.

RESTLESS LEGS SYNDROME

Features
The urge to move legs accompanied by unpleasant sensation in the legs, characterized by relief with movement, aggravation with inactivity, and only occurring or worsening in the evening.

Epidemiology
- Prevalence is 2–7% in the general population.
- Females 1.5–2 times more likely than males.
- Prevalence may be lower in Asian population.

Risk Factors
- Increases with age.
- Strong familial component.
- Iron deficiency.
- Antidepressants, antipsychotics, dopamine-blocking antiemetics, and antihistamines can contribute to or worsen symptoms.
- Multiple medical comorbidities, including cardiovascular disease.

Treatment
- Behavioral strategies including regular exercise, reduced caffeine intake, and avoiding aggravating factors have been shown to be beneficial.
- Responds well to pharmacologic treatments.
- Remove offending agents if possible.
- Iron replacement if low ferritin.
- Dopamine agonists and benzodiazepines are first-line treatments.
- Gabapentin, gabapentin enacarbil (prodrug to gabapentin), and pregablin are also used.
- Low-potency opioids can be used for treatment-refractory patients.

SUBSTANCE/MEDICATION-INDUCED SLEEP DISORDER

- Severe sleep disorder due to substance intoxication/withdrawal or medication.
- Sleep disturbance not better explained by another sleep disorder (e.g., symptoms don't last longer than 1 month after intoxication or withdrawal).
- Can be insomnia, daytime sleepiness, parasomnia, or mixed type.
- Treatment would be to remove the offending substance, or reduce, discontinue, or switch medications (if clinically appropriate).

CHAPTER 16

SEXUAL DYSFUNCTIONS AND PARAPHILIC DISORDERS

Sexual Response Cycle — 174
Sexual Changes with Aging — 174
Differential Diagnosis of Sexual Dysfunctions — 174
Sexual Dysfunctions — 175
Treatment of Sexual Disorders — 176
    Sex Therapy — 176
    Cognitive-Behavioral Therapy — 177
    Hypnosis — 177
    Group Therapy — 177
    Analytically Oriented (Psychodynamic) Psychotherapy — 177
    Pharmacologic Treatment — 177
    Mechanical Therapies — 177
Gender Dysphoria — 178
    Diagnosis and DSM-5 Criteria — 178
    Treatment — 178
Paraphilias — 178
    Examples of Paraphilic Disorders — 179

Sexual dysfunctions include clinically significant disturbances in individuals' ability to respond sexually or to experience sexual pleasure.

Sexual Response Cycle

There are several stages of normal sexual response in men and women:

1. **Desire:** The motivation or interest in sexual activity, often reflected by sexual fantasies.
2. **Excitement/Arousal:** Begins with either fantasy or physical contact. It is characterized by erections and testicular enlargement in men and by vaginal lubrication, clitoral erection, labial swelling, and elevation of the uterus in the pelvis (*tenting*) in women. Both men and women experience flushing, nipple erection, and increased respiration, pulse, and blood pressure.
3. **Orgasm:** In men just prior there is tightening of the scrotal sac and secretion of a few drops of seminal fluid. Women experience contraction of the outer one-third of the vagina and enlargement of the upper one-third of the vagina.
   Men ejaculate and women have contractions of the uterus and lower one-third of the vagina. There is facial grimacing, release of tension, slight clouding of consciousness, involuntary anal sphincter contractions, and acute increase in blood pressure and pulse in both men and women.
4. **Resolution:** Muscles relax and cardiovascular state returns to baseline. Detumescence of genitalia in both sexes. Men have a *refractory period* lasting minutes to hours during which they cannot reexperience orgasm; women have little or no refractory period.

Sexual Changes with Aging

The desire for sexual activity does not usually change as people age. However, men usually require more direct stimulation of genitals and more time to achieve orgasm, with less reliable/strong erections. The intensity of ejaculation usually decreases, and the length of refractory period increases.

After menopause, women experience vaginal dryness and thinning due to decreased levels of estrogen and lubrication. They may also have decreased libido and reduced nipple/clitoral/vulvar sensitivity. These conditions can be treated with hormone replacement therapy or vaginal creams.

Differential Diagnosis of Sexual Dysfunctions

Problems with sexual functioning may be due to any of the following:

- Medical conditions: Examples include atherosclerosis (causing erectile dysfunction from vascular occlusion), diabetes (causing erectile dysfunction from vascular changes and peripheral neuropathy), and pelvic adhesions (causing dyspareunia in women).
- Medication side effects: Antihypertensives, anticholinergics, antidepressants (especially selective serotonin reuptake inhibitors [SSRIs]), and antipsychotics may contribute to sexual dysfunctions.
- Depression.
- Substance use.
- Abnormal levels of gonadal hormones:
  - **Estrogen:** Decreased levels after menopause cause vaginal dryness and thinning in women (without affecting desire).

WARDS TIP

Alcohol and marijuana enhance sexual desire by suppressing inhibitions. However, long-term alcohol use decreases sexual desire. Cocaine and amphetamines enhance libido by stimulating dopamine receptors. Narcotics inhibit libido.

- **Testosterone:** Promotes libido (desire) in both men and women.
- **Progesterone:** May inhibit libido in both men and women by blocking androgen receptors; found in oral contraceptives, hormone replacement therapy, and, occasionally, treatments for prostate cancer.
- Presence of a sexual dysfunction (see below).

Sexual Dysfunctions

Sexual dysfunctions are problems involving any stage of the sexual response cycle. They all share the following *Diagnostic and Statistical Manual of Mental Disorders*, 5th ed. (DSM-5) criteria:

- The disorder causes clinically significant distress.
- The dysfunction is not better explained by a nonsexual mental disorder, as a consequence of severe relationship distress or other stressors, and not attributable to the effects of a substance/medication or another medical condition.

> Mr. Jones is a 58-year-old married man with a history of major depressive disorder who arrives at your outpatient clinic for a yearly follow-up visit. He complains of recent marital problems with his wife of 30 years. He is being treated with an SSRI, and his depressive symptoms have been stable for over 3 years on his current dose. Upon further questioning, he reveals that he has been having sex with his wife less often than usual, "only once or twice a month." He states that this is a marked decrease since his last visit with you. He feels that lately they have been arguing more and feels that their decrease in sexual activity has adversely affected their relationship. He also reports a mild decrease in his energy.
>
> Mr. Jones denies having urges to masturbate in the times between sexual intercourse with his wife. He also denies having any affairs, laughing nervously while saying, "I can barely satisfy my own wife." He appears sad and states that he is beginning to feel "down" about this. When he does have sex, he reports that it is initiated by his wife, and he is initially reluctant to engage in sexual activity. However, once he does, he denies any problems with having or sustaining an erection and denies any difficulties in reaching orgasm. Mr. Jones reports that he drinks two or three drinks per day on the weekends, and he does not use any recreational drugs.
>
> ***What is his most likely diagnosis? What other considerations should be made?***
>
> The patient's most likely diagnosis is male hypoactive sexual desire disorder. Although decreased sexual interest is more prevalent in women, it should not be overlooked in men. As this clinical case shows, the patient does not seem to fantasize or desire sexual activity despite prior history of doing so. He appears distressed by this and reports that it is causing interpersonal dysfunction. Although his depression has remained stable during the past 3 years and the patient does not report symptoms that would suggest a current depressive episode, his sexual complaints and fatigue symptoms might suggest a relapse of depressive symptoms and should be monitored closely. It is also very important to consider if his treatment with an SSRI is affecting his sexual functioning.

KEY FACT

Dopamine enhances libido. Serotonin inhibits sexual function.

WARDS TIP

Causes of sexual dysfunctions may be physiological, psychological, or both. Psychological causes of sexual dysfunctions are often comorbid with other psychiatric disorders, such as depression or anxiety.

WARDS TIP

Problems with sexual desire may be due to stress, relationship difficulties or conflict, poor self-esteem, or unconscious fears about sex.

What should you consider in the initial management of this patient's complaints?

His initial management should consist of a thorough history, a physical examination, and laboratory tests (complete metabolic profile, testosterone levels, thyroid-stimulating hormone levels) that might rule out medical (e.g., endocrine) abnormalities. If another medical disorder, mental disorder, or substance is believed responsible, treatment considerations should include outpatient psychotherapy, sex therapy, cognitive-behavioral therapy, or group therapy.

> **KEY FACT**
>
> The most common sexual dysfunctions in men are erectile disorder and premature ejaculation. The most common in women are female sexual interest/arousal disorder and female orgasmic disorder.

- **Male hypoactive sexual desire disorder:** Absence or deficiency of sexual thoughts, desire, or fantasies for more than 6 months (occurs in 5% of men).
- **Female sexual interest/arousal disorder:** Absence or reduced sexual interest, thoughts/fantasies, initiation of sex, sexual excitement/pleasure, sexual arousal, and/or genital/nongenital sensations during sex for more than 6 months (unclear prevalence of DSM-5 disorder, but low sexual desire in up to 26–43% of women).
- **Erectile disorder:** Marked difficulty obtaining or maintaining an erection, or marked decreased in erectile rigidity for more than 6 months. Commonly referred to as *erectile dysfunction (ED)* or *impotence*. May be *lifelong* (always had difficulty) or *acquired* (after previous ability to maintain erections). ED is the most common sexual disorder in men, with an overall prevalence of approximately 16%.
- **Premature (early) ejaculation:** Recurrent pattern of ejaculation during sex within 1 minute and before the individual wishes it for more than 6 months. Four percent of the population have the disorder, but up to 30% of men report concerns about how rapidly they ejaculate.
- **Female orgasmic disorder:** Marked delay in infrequency/absence/reduced intensity of orgasm for more than 6 months. The prevalence ranges from 20% to 40%.
- **Delayed ejaculation:** Marked delay in infrequency/absence of ejaculation for more than 6 months. Estimated prevalence likely less than 1%.
- **Genito-pelvic pain/penetration disorder:** Persistent or recurrent difficulties in one of the following: vaginal penetration during intercourse, marked vulvovaginal or pelvic pain during intercourse or penetration, marked anticipatory fear or anxiety about vulvovaginal or pelvic pain, or marked tensing or tightening of pelvic floor muscles during attempted vaginal penetration for more than 6 months. Prevalence unknown but up to 27% of American women complain of pain during intercourse. Controversial whether prior sexual/physical abuse or religious orthodoxy predispose.

> **KEY FACT**
>
> Other DSM-5 categories of sexual dysfunction include substance/medication-induced sexual dysfunction and other specified/unspecified sexual dysfunction.

Treatment of Sexual Disorders

SEX THERAPY

Sex therapy utilizes the concept of the couple, rather than the individual, as the target of therapy. Couples meet with a therapist together in sessions to identify and discuss their sexual problems. The therapist recommends sexual exercises for the couple to attempt at home; activities initially focus on heightening sensory awareness (sensate focus exercises) and progressively incorporate increased levels of sexual contact. Treatment is short term. This therapy is most useful when no other psychopathology is involved.

COGNITIVE-BEHAVIORAL THERAPY

Cognitive-behavioral therapy (CBT) approaches sexual dysfunction as a learned maladaptive behavior. It utilizes traditional therapies such as cognitive restructuring, partner communication training, systematic desensitization, and exposure, where patients are progressively exposed to increasing levels of stimuli that provoke their anxiety. Eventually, patients are able to respond appropriately to the stimuli. Other forms of therapy may include muscle relaxation techniques, assertiveness training, and prescribed sexual exercises to try at home. It is also a short-term therapy.

HYPNOSIS

Most often used adjunctively with other therapies. More useful if anxiety is present.

GROUP THERAPY

May be used as a primary or adjunctive therapy.

ANALYTICALLY ORIENTED (PSYCHODYNAMIC) PSYCHOTHERAPY

Individual, long-term therapy that focuses on feelings, past relationships (including familial), fears, fantasies, dreams, and interpersonal problems that may be contributing to sexual disorder.

PHARMACOLOGIC TREATMENT

- **Erectile disorder:** Phosphodiesterase-5 inhibitors (e.g., sildenafil) are given orally, which enhance blood flow to the penis; they require psychological or physical stimulation to achieve an erection. Alprostadil, either injected into the corpora cavernosa or transurethral, acts locally; it produces an erection within 2 to 3 minutes and works in the absence of sexual stimulation.
- **Premature ejaculation:** SSRIs and tricyclic antidepressants (TCAs) prolong the time from stimulation to orgasm.
- **Male hypoactive sexual desire disorder/female sexual interest/arousal disorder:** Testosterone is used as replacement therapy for men with low levels. Low doses may also improve libido in women, especially in postmenopausal women. Low-dose vaginal estrogen replacement may improve vaginal dryness and atrophy in postmenopausal women.

MECHANICAL THERAPIES

- **Erectile disorder:** Vacuum-assisted erection devices, penile prostheses, or surgical insertion of semirigid or inflatable tubes into the corpora cavernosa (used only for end-stage impotence).
- **Female orgasmic disorder:** Directed masturbation (education and self-awareness exercises to reach orgasm through self-stimulation).
- **Premature ejaculation:**
    - The *squeeze technique* is used to increase the threshold of excitability. When the man is excited to near ejaculation, he or his sexual partner

is instructed to squeeze the glans of his penis in order to prevent ejaculation. Gradually, he gains awareness about his sexual sensations and learns to achieve greater ejaculatory control.
- The *stop-start technique* involves cessation of all penile stimulation when the man is near ejaculation. This technique functions in the same manner as the squeeze technique.
- **Genito-pelvic pain/penetration disorder:** Gradual desensitization to achieve intercourse, starting with muscle relaxation techniques, progressing to erotic massage, and finally achieving sexual intercourse.

Gender Dysphoria

Gender dysphoria is commonly referred to as *gender identity disorder, transgender,* or *transsexuality*. Individuals have **distress** accompanying the incongruence between their expressed gender and assigned gender. They may dress as the opposite sex, take sex hormones, or undergo sex change operations.

Cross-gender behaviors in children with this disorder often begin around age 3, the time when gender identity is established. Adults in whom the disorder is first diagnosed usually have experienced some feelings of gender discomfort from early childhood, although the history is not always clear.

Gender dysphoria is often associated with psychological comorbidities such as major depression, anxiety disorders, and suicide. In addition, these individuals are not infrequently the target of harassment and violence.

DIAGNOSIS AND DSM-5 CRITERIA

- **At least two of the following:**
    - A marked incongruence between one's experienced gender and primary/secondary sex characteristics.
    - A strong desire to be rid of one's primary/secondary sex characteristics because of the above.
    - A strong desire for the primary/secondary sex characteristics of the other gender.
    - A strong desire to be of the other gender.
    - A strong desire to be treated as the other gender.
    - A strong conviction that one has the typical feelings/reactions of the other gender.
- Clinically significant distress or impairment in functioning.

TREATMENT

Therapy and family involvement for younger patients; surgical sex reassignment after living 1 year in the desired gender role and after 1 year of continuous hormone therapy.

KEY FACT

Transsexuals identify themselves more with the opposite (of their assigned) gender and commonly undergo surgery to physically appear like the opposite (of their assigned) gender.

Paraphilias

Paraphilic disorders are characterized by engagement in unusual sexual activities and/or preoccupation with unusual sexual urges or fantasies for at least 6 months that either are acted on with a nonconsenting person or cause significant distress or impairment in functioning. Paraphilic fantasies alone are not considered disorders unless they are intense, recurrent, and interfere with daily life; occasional fantasies are considered normal components of sexuality (even if unusual).

Only a small percentage of people suffer from paraphilic disorders. Most paraphilic disorders occur almost exclusively in men, but sadism, masochism, and pedophilia may also occur in women. Voyeuristic and pedophilic disorders are the most common paraphilic disorders.

EXAMPLES OF PARAPHILIC DISORDERS

- **Pedophilic disorder:** Sexual fantasies/urges/behaviors involving sexual acts with prepubescent children (age 13 years or younger). DSM-5 specifies that the person is at least age 16 and at least 5 years older than the child.
- **Frotteuristic disorder:** Sexual arousal from touching or rubbing against a nonconsenting person.
- **Voyeuristic disorder:** Sexual arousal from observing an unsuspecting nude, or disrobing individual (often with binoculars).
- **Exhibitionistic disorder:** Sexual arousal from exposure of one's genitals to an unsuspecting person.
- **Sexual masochism disorder:** Sexual arousal from the act of being humiliated, beaten, bound, or made to suffer.
- **Sexual sadism disorder:** Sexual arousal from the physical or psychological suffering of another person.
- **Fetishistic disorder:** Sexual arousal from either the use of nonliving objects (e.g., shoes or pantyhose) or nongenital body parts.
- **Transvestic disorder:** Sexual arousal from cross-dressing (e.g., wearing women's clothing such as underwear).

Course and Prognosis

- *Poor prognostic factors* are having multiple paraphilias, early age of onset, comorbid substance use, high frequency of behavior, and referral by law enforcement agencies (i.e., after an arrest).
- *Good prognostic factors* are having only one paraphilia, self-referral for treatment, sense of guilt associated with the behavior, and history of otherwise normal sexual activity in addition to the paraphilia.

Treatment

- Difficult to treat.
- Psychotropic medication if associated with a comorbid psychiatric illness.
- Although controversial, antiandrogens, long-acting gonadotropin-releasing hormones, SSRIs, and naltrexone have been used to decrease sex drive and fantasies.
- Cognitive-behavioral therapy can be used to disrupt learned patterns and modify behavior.
- Social skills training.
- Twelve-step programs.
- Group therapy.
- Insight-oriented therapy has been used with questionable benefit.

KEY FACT

The three most common types of paraphilia: pedophilia, voyeurism, exhibitionism.

KEY FACT

Patients often have more than one paraphilia.

KEY FACT

An example of fetishistic disorder is a man being primarily sexually aroused by women's shoes causing significant distress and marital problems.

KEY FACT

An example of transvestic disorder is a person significantly distressed but being sexually aroused by dressing up as a member of the opposite gender. This is not the same as homosexuality or gender dysphoria.

KEY FACT

Most rape offenders are relatives of the victim.

CHAPTER 17

PSYCHOTHERAPIES

Psychoanalysis and Related Therapies	182
Freud's Theories of the Mind	182
TOPOGRAPHIC THEORY	182
STRUCTURAL THEORY	182
Defense Mechanisms	182
MATURE DEFENSES	183
NEUROTIC DEFENSES	183
IMMATURE DEFENSES	184
OTHER DEFENSE MECHANISMS	184
Psychoanalysis	184
IMPORTANT CONCEPTS AND TECHNIQUES USED IN PSYCHOANALYSIS	185
PSYCHOANALYSIS-RELATED THERAPIES	185
Behavioral Therapy	186
LEARNING THEORY	186
CONDITIONING	186
BEHAVIORAL THERAPY TECHNIQUES (DECONDITIONING)	186
Cognitive Therapy	187
CLINICAL EXAMPLE OF THE COGNITIVE THEORY OF DEPRESSION	187
Cognitive-Behavioral Therapy (CBT)	187
Dialectical Behavioral Therapy (DBT)	188
Group Therapy	188
Family Therapy	189
Couples Therapy	189

It is common to combine psychotherapy with medications. *Split treatment* describes the arrangement where a physician prescribes medication and someone else provides therapy. In these cases the physician and therapist should regularly communicate regarding the patient's treatment.

Psychoanalysis and Related Therapies

Psychoanalysis and its related therapies are derived from Sigmund Freud's psychoanalytic theories of the mind. Freud proposed that behaviors, or symptoms, result from *unconscious* mental processes, including defense mechanisms and conflicts between one's ego, id, superego, and external reality. Since the time of Freud, many other psychoanalytic theories have been developed. Influential theorists have included Melanie Klein, Heinz Kohut, Michael Balint, Margaret Mahler, and others.

Examples of psychoanalytic therapies include the following:

- Psychoanalysis.
- Psychoanalytically oriented psychotherapy.
- Brief dynamic therapy.
- Interpersonal therapy.

Freud's Theories of the Mind

TOPOGRAPHIC THEORY

1. **Unconscious:** Includes repressed thoughts that are out of one's awareness; involves *primary process* thinking (primitive, pleasure-seeking urges with no regard to logic or time, prominent in children and psychosis). Thoughts and ideas may be repressed into the unconscious because they are embarrassing, shameful, or otherwise too painful.
2. **Preconscious:** Contains memories that are easy to bring into awareness, but not unless consciously retrieved.
3. **Conscious:** Involves current thoughts and secondary process thinking (logical, organized, mature, and can delay gratification).

STRUCTURAL THEORY

1. **Id:** Unconscious; involves instinctual sexual/aggressive urges and primary process thinking.
2. **Superego:** Moral conscience and ego ideal (inner image of oneself that one wants to become).
3. **Ego:** Serves as a mediator between the id, superego, and external environment, and seeks to develop satisfying interpersonal relationships; uses *defense mechanisms* (see below) to control instinctual urges and distinguishes fantasy from reality using *reality testing*. Problems with reality testing occur in psychotic individuals.

Defense Mechanisms

Defense mechanisms are used by the ego to protect oneself and relieve anxiety by keeping conflicts out of awareness. They are (mostly) *unconscious* processes that are normal and healthy if they are mature in nature and used

> **KEY FACT**
>
> Normal development: Id is present at birth, ego develops after birth, and superego development is traditionally considered to be completed by age 6.

> **KEY FACT**
>
> According to Freud, the superego is the aspect of one's psyche that represents "morality, society, and parental teaching."

> **KEY FACT**
>
> The Freudian superego represents internalization of cultural rules.

> **KEY FACT**
>
> Planning the workday, negotiating traffic, and running a meeting are examples of "executive functioning."

in moderation (i.e., adaptive). They may be unhealthy if immature (i.e., maladaptive). Immature defense mechanisms can be used excessively as seen in some psychiatric disorders.

Defense mechanisms are often classified hierarchically. **Mature** defense mechanisms are healthy and adaptive, and they are seen in normal adults. **Neurotic** defenses are encountered in obsessive-compulsive patients, patients with other anxiety disorders, and adults under stress. **Immature** defenses are seen in children, adolescents, psychotic patients, and some nonpsychotic patients, such as patients with severe personality disorders. They are the most primitive defense mechanisms.

MATURE DEFENSES

Mature ego defenses are commonly found in healthy, high-functioning adults. These defenses often help people integrate conflicting emotions and thoughts.

1. **Altruism:** Performing acts that benefit others in order to vicariously experience pleasure. (*Clinical example:* A patient's child recently died from ovarian cancer. As part of the grieving process, the patient donates money to help raise community awareness about the symptoms of ovarian cancer so other patients could potentially benefit from early intervention.)
2. **Humor:** Expressing (usually) unpleasant or uncomfortable feelings without causing discomfort to self or others.
3. **Sublimation:** Satisfying socially objectionable impulses in an acceptable manner (thus *channeling* them rather than *preventing* them). (*Clinical example:* Person with unconscious urges to physically control others becomes a prison guard.)
4. **Suppression:** Purposely ignoring an unacceptable impulse or emotion in order to diminish discomfort and accomplish a task. (*Clinical example:* Nurse who feels nauseated by an infected wound puts aside feelings of disgust to clean wound and provide necessary patient care.)

> **KEY FACT**
>
> Suppression, as a defense mechanism, is a *conscious* process that involves avoiding paying attention to a particular emotion. Therefore, it is not an unconscious process.

 A former street thug becomes a social worker to help reform kids in gangs. *What is the defense mechanism?* Sublimation—the channeling of destructive impulses to create something constructive.

NEUROTIC DEFENSES

1. **Controlling:** Regulating situations and events of external environment to relieve anxiety.
2. **Displacement:** Shifting emotions from an undesirable situation to one that is personally tolerable. (*Clinical example:* Student who is angry with his mother talks back to his teacher the next day and refuses to obey her instructions.)
3. **Intellectualization:** Avoiding negative feelings by excessive use of intellectual functions and by focusing on irrelevant details. (*Clinical example:* Physician dying from colon cancer describes the pathophysiology of his disease in detail to his 12-year-old son.)
4. **Isolation of affect:** Unconsciously limiting the experience of feelings or emotions associated with a stressful life event in order to avoid anxiety. (*Clinical example:* Woman describes the recent death of her beloved husband without emotion.)

KEY FACT

Intellectualization is a defense mechanism where reasoning is used to block confrontation with an unconscious conflict or undesirable thought or feeling.

5. **Rationalization:** Explanations of an event to justify outcomes or behaviors and to make them acceptable. (*Clinical example:* "My boss fired me today because she's not meeting her quotas, not because I haven't done a good job.")
6. **Reaction formation:** Doing the opposite of an unacceptable impulse. (*Clinical example:* Man who is in love with his married coworker insults her.)
7. **Repression:** Preventing a thought or feeling from entering consciousness. (Repression is unconscious, whereas suppression is a conscious act.)

> A man buys himself an expensive new watch and tells his friends that he needed it because his old one was not reliable enough and he needs to make sure to get to his appointments on time. *Think: Rationalization.*

IMMATURE DEFENSES

1. **Acting out:** Giving in to an impulse, even if socially inappropriate, in order to avoid the anxiety of suppressing that impulse. (*Clinical example:* Man who has been told his therapist is going on vacation "forgets" his last appointment and skips it.)
2. **Denial:** Not accepting reality that is too painful. (*Clinical example:* Woman who has been scheduled for a breast mass biopsy cancels her appointment because she believes she is healthy.)
3. **Regression:** Performing behaviors from an earlier stage of development in order to avoid tension associated with current phase of development. (*Clinical example:* Woman brings her childhood teddy bear to the hospital when she has to spend the night.)
4. **Projection:** Attributing objectionable thoughts or emotions to others. (*Clinical example:* Husband who is attracted to other women believes his wife is having an affair.)

KEY FACT

A man who accuses his wife of cheating on him while involved in numerous affairs is an example of projection.

OTHER DEFENSE MECHANISMS

1. **Splitting:** Labeling people as all good or all bad; often seen in borderline personality disorder. (*Clinical example:* Woman who tells her doctor, "You and the nurses are the only people who understand me; all the other doctors are mean and impatient.")
2. **Undoing:** Attempting to reverse a situation by adopting a new behavior. (*Clinical example:* Man who has had a brief fantasy of killing his wife by sabotaging her car takes the car in for a complete checkup.)

WARDS TIP

Be on guard when your patient thinks you're so cool to talk to but hates the "evil attending." That's splitting.

Psychoanalysis

The goal of psychoanalysis is to resolve *unconscious conflicts* by bringing repressed experiences and feelings into awareness and integrating them into the patient's conscious experience. Psychoanalysis is therefore considered *insight oriented.* Patients best suited for psychoanalysis have the following characteristics: not psychotic, intelligent, and stable in relationships and daily living. Treatment is usually 3 to 5 days per week for many years. During therapy sessions, the patient usually lies on a couch with the therapist seated out of view.

To become an analyst, professionals (MDs, PhDs, PsyDs, and MSWs) must complete training at a psychoanalytic institute. In addition to attending seminars and treating patients under supervision, the training requires that they receive their own analysis.

Psychoanalysis can be useful in the treatment of the following:

- Clusters B and C personality disorders.
- Anxiety disorders.
- Problems coping with life events.
- Sexual disorders.
- Persistent depressive disorder.

WARDS TIP

Psychoanalysis is not indicated for people who have problems with reality testing, such as actively psychotic or manic patients.

IMPORTANT CONCEPTS AND TECHNIQUES USED IN PSYCHOANALYSIS

- **Free association:** The patient is asked to say whatever comes into his or her mind during therapy sessions. The purpose is to bring forth thoughts and feelings from the unconscious so that the therapist may interpret them.
- **Dream interpretation:** Dreams are seen to represent conflict between urges and fears. Interpretation of dreams by the psychoanalyst is used to help achieve therapeutic goals.
- **Therapeutic alliance:** This is the bond between the therapist and the patient, who work together toward a therapeutic goal.
- **Transference:** Projection of unconscious feelings regarding important figures in the patient's life onto the therapist. Interpretation of transference is used to help the patient gain insight and resolve unconscious conflict.
- **Countertransference:** Projection of unconscious feelings about important figures in the therapist's life onto the patient. The therapist must remain aware of countertransference issues, as they may interfere with his or her objectivity.

KEY FACT

An example of transference would be when a patient who has repressed feelings of abandonment by her father becomes angry when her therapist is late for the appointment.

PSYCHOANALYSIS-RELATED THERAPIES

Examples of psychoanalysis-related therapies include:

1. **Psychoanalytically oriented psychotherapy** and **brief dynamic psychotherapy:** These employ similar techniques and theories as psychoanalysis, but they are less frequent, less intense, usually briefer (weekly sessions for 6 months to several years), and involve face-to-face sessions between the therapist and patient (no couch).
2. **Interpersonal therapy:** Attachment-focused psychotherapy that centers on the development of skills to help treat certain psychiatric disorders. Treatment is brief (once-weekly sessions for 3 to 4 months). The idea is to improve interpersonal relations. Sessions focus on reassurance, clarification of emotions, improving interpersonal communication, and testing perceptions. It has demonstrated efficacy in the treatment of depression and has been modified for use in adolescents.
3. **Supportive psychotherapy:** Purpose is to help patient feel safe during a difficult time and help to build up the patient's healthy defenses. Treatment is not insight oriented but instead focuses on empathy, understanding, and education. Supportive therapy is commonly used as adjunctive treatment in even the most severe mental disorders.

Behavioral Therapy

Behavioral therapy, pioneered by B. F. Skinner, seeks to treat psychiatric disorders by helping patients change behaviors that contribute to their symptoms. It can be used to extinguish maladaptive behaviors (such as phobic avoidance, compulsions, etc.) by replacing them with healthy alternatives. The time course is usually brief, and it is almost always combined with cognitive therapy as CBT.

LEARNING THEORY

Behavioral therapy is based on **learning theory,** which states that behaviors are learned by *conditioning* and can similarly be unlearned by *deconditioning*.

CONDITIONING

- **Classical conditioning:** A stimulus can evoke a conditioned response. (*Example:* Pavlov's dog would salivate when hearing a bell because the dog had learned that bells were always followed by food.)
- **Operant conditioning:** Behaviors can be learned when followed by positive or negative *reinforcement.* (*Example:* Skinner box—a rat presses a lever by accident and receives food; eventually, it learns to press the lever for food [trial-and-error learning].)

BEHAVIORAL THERAPY TECHNIQUES (DECONDITIONING)

- **Systematic desensitization:** The patient performs relaxation techniques while being exposed to increasing doses of an anxiety-provoking stimulus. Gradually, he or she learns to use relaxation skills to tolerate and cope with the anxiety provoking stimulus. Commonly used to treat phobic disorders. (*Example:* A patient who has a fear of spiders is first shown a photograph of a spider, followed by exposure to a stuffed toy spider, then a videotape of a spider, and finally a live spider. At each step, the patient learns to relax while exposed to an increasing dose of the phobia.)
- **Flooding and implosion:** Through habituation, the patient is confronted with a real (flooding) or imagined (implosion) anxiety-provoking stimulus and not allowed to withdraw from it until he or she feels calm and in control. Relaxation exercises are used to help the patient tolerate the stimulus. Less commonly used than systematic desensitization to treat phobic disorders. (*Example:* A patient who has a fear of flying is made to fly in an airplane [flooding] or imagine flying [implosion].)
- **Aversion therapy:** A negative stimulus (such as an electric shock) is repeatedly paired with a specific behavior to create an unpleasant response. Used to treat addictions or paraphilic disorders. (*Example:* An alcoholic patient is prescribed Antabuse, which makes him ill every time he drinks alcohol.)
- **Token economy:** Rewards are given after specific behaviors to positively reinforce them. Commonly used to encourage showering, shaving, and other positive behaviors in disorganized patients. Also frequently used in treatment of substance use disorders on rehabilitation units as part of a contingency management program where abstinence is reinforced with material rewards or privileges.
- **Biofeedback:** Physiological data (such as heart rate and blood pressure measurements) are given to patients as they try to mentally control physiological states. Can be used to treat anxiety disorders, migraines,

---

KEY FACT

Positive reinforcement: Giving a reward for a desired behavior.

KEY FACT

Negative reinforcement: Encouraging a behavior by removing an aversive stimulus. (*Example*: Putting on the seatbelt in the car in order to stop the beeping.) Punishment, in contrast, is an aversive response to a behavior. Punishment is *not* negative reinforcement.

hypertension, chronic pain, asthma, and incontinence. (*Example:* A patient is given her heart rate and blood pressure measurements during a migraine while being instructed to mentally control visceral changes that affect her pain.)

KEY FACT

Biofeedback used to treat a wide scope of clinical conditions including agoraphobia, fecal incontinence, tension headache, and hypertension.

Cognitive Therapy

Cognitive therapy, pioneered by Aaron T. Beck, seeks to correct faulty assumptions and negative feelings that exacerbate psychiatric symptoms. The patient is taught to identify maladaptive thoughts and replace them with positive ones. It is most commonly used to treat depressive and anxiety disorders, and is usually combined with behavioral therapy in CBT. May also be used for paranoid personality disorder, obsessive-compulsive disorder, somatic symptom disorders, and eating disorders. Cognitive therapy can be as effective as medication for some disorders.

CLINICAL EXAMPLE OF THE COGNITIVE THEORY OF DEPRESSION

- **Cognitive distortions,** also known as **faulty assumptions** or **automatic thoughts**. (*Example:* If I were smart, I would do well on tests. I must not be smart since I received average grades this semester.)
- **Negative thoughts.** (*Example:* I am stupid. I will never amount to anything worthwhile. Nobody likes a worthless person.)

Cognitive-Behavioral Therapy (CBT)

CBT combines theories and approaches from cognitive therapy and behavior therapy. Treatment follows a protocol or manual with homework assignments between therapy sessions. During therapy sessions, the patient and therapist set an **agenda,** review homework, and challenge cognitive distortions. The patients learn how their feelings and behavior are influenced by their thoughts. Treatment is usually brief and may last from 6 weeks to 6 months. Research has shown that CBT is effective for many psychiatric illnesses, including depression, anxiety disorders, schizophrenia, and substance use disorders.

 Mrs. Ramos is a 22-year-old college student who is hospitalized after she tried to kill herself by taking an overdose of fluoxetine. This is her fifth overdose, and all have been in response to perceived rejections. She often feels "empty inside" and reports that she has had many intense relationships that have ended abruptly. She reports that she has been married for 1 year but fights constantly with her husband because of suspicions that he is unfaithful. Her husband denies these allegations and reports that he is tired of her outbursts, explaining that she yells at him and has become physically abusive. He has threatened to divorce her if these behaviors continue. During your evaluation, you notice multiple healed scars over her forearms, and she admits to self-harm behavior by cutting and burning herself because, "When I get angry, it helps me feel better."

During her hospitalization, you notice that her mood has improved and that she has become close to other patients. She says, "They are like family." Although you have seen her only twice, she thinks you are "a great doctor," unlike the psychiatrists who have treated her in the past, who have all been "idiots." You call her outpatient therapist, who confirms that she has been diagnosed with borderline personality disorder.

What are the recommended psychotherapeutic modalities for this patient?

Dialectical behavioral therapy (DBT) and psychoanalytic/psychodynamic therapy have shown to be effective treatments in randomized controlled trials for borderline personality disorder. DBT is a form of cognitive-behavioral therapy that is effective in reducing the urges to engage in self-harm behavior and leads to fewer hospital days. Although the efficacy of couples therapy in borderline patients has been debated, it might be considered in this case.

What special considerations should be taken into account when engaging in psychotherapy?

The psychotherapist should always be aware of positive or negative countertransference developed toward the patient. Frequent discussion and counseling with colleagues is useful. Patients with borderline personality disorder are challenging to treat due to their intense emotions, impulsivity, and anger.

What particular defense mechanism is exhibited by Mrs. Ramos?

Mrs. Ramos exhibits splitting as evidenced by her extreme dichotomous thinking in expressing that you are a "great" psychiatrist, whereas other psychiatrists who have treated her in the past are "idiots."

WARDS TIP

CBT focuses on a patient's current symptoms and problems by examining the connection between thoughts, feelings, and behaviors.

Dialectical Behavioral Therapy (DBT)

DBT was developed by Marsha Linehan, and its effectiveness has been demonstrated in research trials. Once-weekly individual and group treatment can effectively diminish the self-destructive behaviors and hospitalizations of patients with borderline personality disorder. It incorporates cognitive and supportive techniques, along with the "mindfulness" derived from traditional Buddhist practice. DBT has demonstrated effectiveness in patients with borderline personality disorders and eating disorders.

Group Therapy

- Three or more patients with a similar problem or pathology meet together with a therapist for group sessions. Many of the psychotherapeutic techniques already reviewed are used, including behavioral, cognitive, and supportive.

- Certain groups are *peer led* (including 12-step groups like Alcoholics Anonymous) and do not have a therapist present to facilitate the group. These groups meet to discuss problems, share feelings, and provide support to each other.
- Group therapy is especially useful in the treatment of substance use disorders, adjustment disorders, and personality disorders. Advantages of group therapy over individual therapy include:
  - Patients get immediate feedback and support from their peers.
  - Patients gain insight into their own condition by listening to others with similar problems.
  - If a therapist is present, there is an opportunity to observe interactions between others who may be eliciting a variety of transferences.

Family Therapy

Family therapy is useful as an adjunctive treatment in many psychiatric conditions because:

1. An individual's problems usually affect the entire family. He or she may be viewed differently and treated differently after the development of psychopathology, and new tensions and conflicts within the family may arise.
2. Psychopathology may arise or worsen due to dysfunction within the family unit. These conditions are most effectively treated with the entire family present. Evidence demonstrates that **high expressed emotion** (critical and emotionally over-involved attitudes toward a family member) negatively impacts mental health in psychiatric patients.

The goals of family therapy are to reduce conflict, help members understand each other's needs *(mutual accommodation)*, and help the family unit cope with internally destructive forces. **Boundaries** between family members may be too rigid or too permeable, and **"triangles"** may result when two family members form an alliance against a third member. The therapist may assist in correcting these problems. (*Example of boundaries that may be too permeable:* A mother and daughter smoke marijuana together and share intimate details about their sexual activities.) Family therapy is especially useful in treating schizophrenia and anorexia in adolescents.

Couples Therapy

Couples therapy is useful in the treatment of conflicts, sexual problems, and communication problems within the context of an intimate relationship. The therapist sees the couple together **(conjoint therapy)**, but they may also be seen separately **(concurrent therapy)**. In addition, each person may have a separate therapist and be seen individually **(collaborative therapy)**. In the treatment of sexual problems, two therapists may see the couple together **(four-way therapy)**. Relative contraindications include lack of motivation by one or both spouses and severe illness in one of the spouses (e.g., schizophrenia).

NOTES

CHAPTER 18

PSYCHOPHARMACOLOGY

Side Effects in a Nutshell	192
Antidepressants	193
Selective Serotonin Reuptake Inhibitors	193
Serotonin-Norepinephrine Reuptake Inhibitors (SNRIs)	195
Miscellaneous Antidepressants	195
Heterocyclic Antidepressants	196
Tricyclic Antidepressants	196
Tetracyclic Antidepressants	196
Monoamine Oxidase Inhibitors	197
Antidepressant Use in Other Disorders	198
Antipsychotics	198
Typical (First-Generation) Antipsychotics	199
Atypical (Second-Generation) Antipsychotics	201
Mood Stabilizers	203
Lithium	203
Anticonvulsants	204
Carbamazepine (Tegretol)	204
Valproic Acid (Depakote and Depakene)	204
Anxiolytics/Hypnotics	205
Benzodiazepines	205
Non-BDZ Hypnotics	206
Non-BDZ Anxiolytics	207
Psychostimulants	207
Cognitive Enhancers	208
Acetylcholinesterase Inhibitors	208
NMDA (Glutamate) Receptor Antagonist	208
Reference List of Medications That May Cause Psychiatric Symptoms	208
Psychosis	208
Agitation/Confusion/Delirium	208
Depression	208
Anxiety	208
Sedation/Poor Concentration	209
Selected Medications	209
Other Treatments	209
Electroconvulsive Therapy (ECT)	209
Deep Brain Stimulation (DBS)	209
Repetitive Transcranial Magnetic Stimulation (rTMS)	209
Light Therapy	210
Ketamine Infusion	210

Side Effects in a Nutshell

1. **HAM side effects** (*antiHistamine*—sedation, weight gain; *antiAdrenergic*—hypotension; *antiMuscarinic (anticholinergic)*—dry mouth, blurred vision, urinary retention, constipation, exacerbation of neurocognitive disorders (i.e., dementias).
   - Found in tricyclic antidepressants (TCAs) and low-potency antipsychotics.
2. **Serotonin syndrome:** Confusion, flushing, diaphoresis, tremor, myoclonic jerks, hyperthermia, hypertonicity, rhabdomyolysis, renal failure, and death.
   - Occurs when there is too much serotonin, classically when selective serotonin reuptake inhibitors (SSRIs) and monoamine oxidase inhibitors (MAOIs) are combined. As this combination is rarely seen in practice anymore, serotonin syndrome is more commonly seen when a patient is prescribed multiple medications with serotonergic activity (e.g., SSRIs/SNRIs, trazodone, Tramadol, triptans, dextromethorphan, St. John's wort, ondansetron).
   - Treatment: Stop medications, supportive care.
3. **Hypertensive crisis:** Caused by a buildup of stored catecholamines; triggered by the combination of MAOIs with tyramine-rich foods (e.g., red wine, cheese, chicken liver, cured meats) or with sympathomimetics.
4. **Extrapyramidal side effects (EPS):** *Parkinsonism*—masklike face, cogwheel rigidity, bradykinesia, pill-rolling tremor; *akathisia*—restlessness, need to move, and agitation; *dystonia*—sustained, painful contraction of muscles of neck, tongue, eyes, diaphragm.
   - Occur more frequently with high-potency, typical (first generation) antipsychotics, but can also be seen with atypical (second generation) antipsychotics.
   - Reversible.
   - Occur within *hours to days* of starting medications or increasing doses.
   - In rare cases, can be life threatening (e.g., dystonia of the diaphragm causing asphyxiation).
5. **Hyperprolactinemia:** Occurs with high-potency, typical (first generation) antipsychotics and risperidone.
6. **Tardive dyskinesia (TD):** Choreoathetoid muscle movements, usually of the mouth and tongue (can affect extremities, as well).
   - Occurs after *years* of antipsychotic use (more likely with high-potency, first-generation antipsychotics).
   - Usually irreversible.
7. **Neuroleptic malignant syndrome:** Mental status changes, fever, tachycardia, hypertension, tremor, elevated creatine phosphokinase (CPK), "lead pipe" rigidity.
   - Can be caused by any antipsychotic after a short or long time (increased with high-potency, typical antipsychotics).
   - A medical emergency with up to a 20% mortality rate.
8. **Drug interactions:** *Cytochrome P450* is a group of enzymes in the liver that metabolizes many common drugs, including psychiatric medications.
   - Some medications *induce* the system, in other words the system metabolizes medications faster—drug levels *decrease*.
   - Some medications *inhibit* the system, in other words the system metabolizes medications more slowly—drug levels *increase*.
   - Common cytochrome P450 enzymes important in metabolizing psychiatric medications include CYP3A4, CYP2D6, CYP1A2, CYP2C9, CYP2C19.

WARDS TIP

Drugs that increase serotonin may be found in over-the-counter medicines (e.g., dextromethorphan, St. John's wort). They can cause serotonin syndrome when taken in high doses or in combination with other serotonergic agents.

KEY FACT

Keeping the "kinesias" (impairment of body function) straight:
- Tardive dyskinesia is characterized by Choreoathetoid movements and tongue protrusion.
- Acute dystonia is characterized by twisting and abnormal postures.
- Akathisia is characterized by the inability to sit still.
- Bradykinesia is characterized by decreased or slow body movement.

KEY FACT

First-generation antipsychotics (typicals) are more associated with EPS and second-generation antipsychotics (atypicals) are more associated with metabolic side effects.

- Important CYP450 *inducers* include:
  - Tobacco (1A2).
  - Carbamazepine (1A2, 2C9, 3A4).
  - Barbiturates (2C9).
  - St. John's wort (2C19, 3A4).
- Important CYP450 *inhibitors* include:
  - Fluvoxamine (1A2, 2C19, 3A4).
  - Fluoxetine (2C19, 2C9, 2D6).
  - Paroxetine (2D6).
  - Duloxetine (2D6).
  - Sertraline (2D6).

Antidepressants

- The major categories of antidepressants are:
  - SSRIs.
  - SNRIs.
  - Heterocyclic antidepressants, including TCAs and tetracyclic antidepressants.
  - MAOIs.
  - Miscellaneous antidepressants.
- All antidepressants have similar response rates in treating major depression but differ in safety and side-effect profiles.
- Approximately 60 to 70% of patients with major depression will respond to an antidepressant medication.
- It usually takes 4 to 6 weeks on a given dose of an antidepressant for a patient to fully benefit from a trial of the medication.
- For patients who are prone to side effects, it's important to start at a low dose and titrate up slowly.
- Many antidepressants have a *withdrawal phenomenon*, characterized by dizziness, headaches, nausea, insomnia, and malaise; depending on the dose and half-life, they may need to be tapered.
- Because of their safety and tolerability, SSRIs and related antidepressants have become the most common agents used to treat major depression. However, the choice of a particular medication used for a given patient should be made based on:
  - Patient's particular symptoms
  - Previous treatment responses by the patient or a family member to a particular medication
  - Side-effect profile
  - Comorbid (medical and psychiatric) conditions
  - Risk of suicide via overdose on the medication
  - Cost

SELECTIVE SEROTONIN REUPTAKE INHIBITORS

- SSRIs inhibit presynaptic serotonin pumps that take up serotonin, leading to increased availability of serotonin in synaptic clefts. Additionally, SSRIs cause downstream effects increasing brain plasticity—this mechanism has been hypothesized to explain the delay to onset of antidepressant effect.
- Although structural differences are minimal, patients often respond differently (in regards to efficacy and side effects) to different SSRIs.
- Based on their half-lives, most SSRIs can be dosed daily. Fluoxetine has a weekly dosing form available, as well.

KEY FACT

The Food and Drug Administration (FDA) has a Black Box Warning for all SSRIs potentially increasing "suicidal thinking and behavior." This warning applies to children and young adults to age 25, but may be accurate for older adults as well.

WARDS TIP

The sexual side effects of SSRIs can be treated by either reducing the dose (if clinically appropriate), changing to a non-SSRI antidepressant, augmenting the regimen with bupropion, or, in men, by adding medications like sildenafil.

WARDS TIP

Patients should receive an adequate trial of antidepressant medication, usually at least 4 to 6 weeks at a full dose, before the medication is deemed non-efficacious.

WARDS TIP

Paroxetine is the SSRI that is most associated with weight gain. Fluoxetine and sertraline are considered the most weight-neutral SSRIs

WARDS TIP

SSRIs can **increase** levels of warfarin, requiring **increased** monitoring when starting and stopping these medications.

KEY FACT

Serotonin syndrome is common when serotonergic drugs are used with MAOIs. SSRIs should not be used for at least 2 weeks before or after use of an MAOI.

- There is no correlation between plasma levels and efficacy or side effects.
- SSRIs are the most commonly prescribed antidepressants due to several distinct advantages:
    - Low incidence of side effects, most of which resolve with time.
    - No food restrictions.
    - Much safer in overdose.
- Examples of SSRIs include:
    - **Fluoxetine (Prozac):**
        - Longest half-life, with active metabolites; therefore, no need to taper.
        - Safe in pregnancy, approved for use in children and adolescents.
        - Common side effects: insomnia, anxiety, sexual dysfunction.
        - Can elevate levels of antipsychotics, leading to increased side effects.
    - **Sertraline (Zoloft):**
        - Higher risk for gastrointestinal (GI) disturbances.
        - Very few drug interactions.
        - Other common side effects: insomnia, anxiety, sexual dysfunction.
    - **Paroxetine (Paxil):**
        - A potent inhibitor of CYP26, which can lead to several drug–drug interactions.
        - Common side effects: anticholinergic effects (e.g., sedation, constipation, weight gain) and sexual dysfunction.
        - Short half-life leading to *withdrawal phenomena* if not taken consistently.
    - **Fluvoxamine (Luvox):**
        - Currently approved only for use in obsessive-compulsive disorder (OCD).
        - Common side effects: nausea and vomiting.
        - Multiple drug interactions due to CYP inhibition.
    - **Citalopram (Celexa):**
        - Fewest drug–drug interactions.
        - Dose-dependent QTc prolongation.
    - **Escitalopram (Lexapro):**
        - Levo-enantiomer of citalopram; similar efficacy, possibly fewer side effects.
        - Dose-dependent QTc prolongation.

Side Effects

- SSRIs have significantly fewer side effects than TCAs and MAOIs due to serotonin selectivity (they do not act on histamine, adrenergic, or muscarinic receptors).
- They are much safer in overdose. Most side effects occur because of the extensive number of serotonin receptors throughout the body, including the GI tract.
- Many of the side effects of SSRIs resolve within a few days to weeks and include:
    - GI disturbance: Mostly nausea and diarrhea; giving with food can help.
    - Insomnia; also vivid dreams, often resolves over time.
    - Headache.
    - Weight changes (up or down).
- Other side effects include:
    - Sexual dysfunction (30–40%): decreased libido, anorgasmia, delayed ejaculation. These may occur weeks to months after taking an SSRI and typically do not resolve.
    - Restlessness: An akathisia-like state.

- **Serotonin syndrome:** Caused by an excess of serotonin in the body. It can result from taking a single serotonergic agent, or by taking multiple serotonergic agents in combination. One example is triptans (for migraine headaches) used with SSRIs. Serotonin syndrome is characterized by fever, diaphoresis, tachycardia, hypertension, delirium, and neuromuscular excitability (especially hyperreflexia and "electric jolt" limb movements), potentially death.
- Hyponatremia: Rare.
- Seizures: Rate of approximately 0.2%, slightly lower than TCAs.

SEROTONIN-NOREPINEPHRINE REUPTAKE INHIBITORS (SNRIs)

- **Venlafaxine (Effexor):**
    - Often used for depressive disorders, anxiety disorders like generalized anxiety disorder (GAD), and neuropathic pain.
    - Low drug interaction potential.
    - Extended release (XR form) allows for once-daily dosing.
    - Side-effect profile similar to SSRIs, with the exception of increased blood pressure (BP) in higher doses; do not use in patients with untreated or labile BP.
    - New form, **desvenlafaxine (Pristiq),** is the active metabolite of venlafaxine; it is expensive and without known benefit over venlafaxine.
- **Duloxetine (Cymbalta):**
    - Often used for people with **depression, neuropathic pain,** and in fibromyalgia.
    - Side effects are similar to SSRIs, but more dry mouth and constipation relating to its norepinephrine effects.
    - Hepatotoxicity may be more likely in patients with liver disease or heavy alcohol use, so liver function tests should be monitored when indicated.

MISCELLANEOUS ANTIDEPRESSANTS

- **Bupropion (Wellbutrin):**
    - Norepinephrine-dopamine reuptake inhibitor.
    - Relative **lack of sexual side effects** as compared to the SSRIs.
    - Some efficacy in treatment of adult attention deficit hyperactivity disorder (ADHD)
    - Effective for smoking cessation.
    - Weight neutral.
    - Side effects include increased anxiety, as well as increased risk of **seizures** and psychosis at high doses.
    - Contraindicated in patients with epilepsy or active eating disorders, and in those currently on an MAOI. Use with caution with agents that also lower the seizure threshold (like stimulants).

Serotonin Receptor Antagonists and Agonists

- **Trazodone (Desyrel)** and **Nefazodone (Serzone):**
    - Useful in the treatment of major depression, major depression with anxiety, and **insomnia** (secondary to its sedative effects).
    - They do not have the sexual side effects of SSRIs and do not affect rapid eye movement (REM) sleep.
    - Side effects include nausea, dizziness, orthostatic hypotension, cardiac arrhythmias, **sedation,** and **priapism** (especially with **trazodone**).
    - Because of orthostatic hypotension in higher doses, trazodone is not frequently used solely as an antidepressant. It is commonly used to

KEY FACT

Wellbutrin (bupropion) is *not* associated with the sexual side effects of other antidepressants.

treat insomnia often when initiating an SSRI (until insomnia improves as the depression resolves).
- Nefazodone carries a **Black Box Warning** for rare but serious liver failure (1 per 250,000–300,000 people) and is rarely used.

α2-Adrenergic Receptor Antagonists

- **Mirtazapine (Remeron):**
  - Useful in the treatment of **major depression,** especially in patients who have significant weight loss and/or insomnia.
  - Side effects include **sedation**, **weight gain,** dizziness, tremor, dry mouth, constipation, and (rarely) agranulocytosis.
  - Fewer sexual side effects compared to SSRIs and few drug interactions.

HETEROCYCLIC ANTIDEPRESSANTS

- TCAs inhibit the reuptake of norepinephrine and serotonin, increasing availability of monoamines in the synapse.
- Because of the long half-lives, most are dosed once daily.
- They are rarely used as first-line agents due to a higher incidence of side effects, titration of dosing, and **lethality in overdose.**

TRICYCLIC ANTIDEPRESSANTS

- **Tertiary amines** (highly anticholinergic/antihistaminergic [more sedating]/antiadrenergic [more orthostasis] with a greater lethality in overdose):
  - **Amitriptyline (Elavil):** Useful in chronic pain, migraines, and insomnia.
  - **Imipramine (Tofranil):**
    - Has intramuscular form.
    - Useful in **enuresis** and panic disorder.
  - **Clomipramine (Anafranil):** Most serotonin-specific, therefore useful in the treatment of **OCD**.
  - **Doxepin (Sinequan):**
    - Useful in treating chronic pain.
    - Emerging use as a sleep aid in low doses.
- **Secondary amines**—metabolites of tertiary amines (less anticholinergic/antihistaminic/antiadrenergic):
  - **Nortriptyline (Pamelor, Aventyl):**
    - Least likely to cause orthostatic hypotension.
    - Useful therapeutic blood levels.
    - Useful in treating chronic pain.
  - **Desipramine (Norpramin):**
    - More activating/least sedating.
    - Least anticholinergic.

TETRACYCLIC ANTIDEPRESSANTS

- **Amoxapine (Asendin):**
  - Metabolite of antipsychotic loxapine.
  - May cause EPS and has a similar side-effect profile to typical antipsychotics.

Side Effects

- TCAs are *highly* protein bound and lipid soluble, and therefore can interact with other medications that have high protein binding.

KEY FACT

Trazodone causes priapism: Remember the phrase "Trazo-bone."

KEY FACT

Mirtazapine (Remeron) is good for treating major depression in the elderly—it helps with both sleep and appetite.

WARDS TIP

A 1-week supply of TCAs (as little as 1–2 g) can be lethal in overdose.

- The side effects of TCAs are mostly due to their lack of specificity and interaction with other receptors.
- Antihistaminic properties: Sedation and weight gain.
- Antiadrenergic properties (**cardiovascular** side effects): Orthostatic hypotension, dizziness, reflex tachycardia, arrhythmias (block cardiac sodium channel), and electrocardiographic (ECG) changes (widening QRS, QT, and PR intervals). Avoid in patients with preexisting conduction abnormalities or recent MI.
- Antimuscarinic effects (also called anticholinergic): Dry mouth, constipation, urinary retention, blurred vision, tachycardia, and exacerbation of narrow angle glaucoma.
- Lethal in overdose—must carefully assess the suicide risk when prescribing. Symptoms of overdose include agitation, tremors, ataxia, arrhythmias, delirium, hypoventilation from central nervous system (CNS) depression, myoclonus, hyperreflexia, seizures, and coma.
- Seizures: Risk of seizure is directly related to the dose and serum level (i.e., higher risk of seizures at high doses and overdoses).
- Serotonergic effects: Erectile/ejaculatory dysfunction in males, anorgasmia in females.

WARDS TIP

The treatment for TCA overdose is IV sodium bicarbonate.

WARDS TIP

Major complications of TCAs—3Cs:
Cardiotoxicity
Convulsions
Coma

KEY FACT

Dry mouth, urinary retention, constipation, and blurry vision are some of the side effects of TCAs, caused by the anticholinergic effects.

MONOAMINE OXIDASE INHIBITORS

- MAOIs prevent the inactivation of biogenic amines such as *norepinephrine*, *serotonin*, *dopamine*, and *tyramine* (an intermediate in the conversion of tyrosine to norepinephrine).
- By **irreversibly** inhibiting the enzymes *MAO-A* and *B*, MAOIs increase the number of neurotransmitters available in synapses.
- MAO-A preferentially deactivates serotonin and norepinephrine, and MAO-B preferentially deactivates phenethylamine; *both* types also act on dopamine and tyramine.
- MAOIs are not used as first-line agents because of the increased safety and tolerability of newer agents, notably SSRIs/SNRIs. However, MAOIs are used for certain types of **refractory depression** and in refractory anxiety disorders:
  - **Phenelzine (Nardil)**.
  - **Tranylcypromine (Parnate)**.
  - **Isocarboxazid (Marplan)**.

Side Effects

- **Serotonin syndrome** occurs when **SSRIs** and **MAOIs** are taken together or if other drugs cause increase in serotonin levels.
  - Initially characterized by lethargy, restlessness, confusion, flushing, diaphoresis, tremor, and myoclonic jerks.
  - May progress to hyperthermia, hypertonicity, rhabdomyolysis, renal failure, convulsions, coma, and death.
  - Wait at least 2 weeks before switching from SSRI to MAOI, and at least 5 to 6 weeks with fluoxetine.
- **Hypertensive crisis:** Risk when MAOIs are taken with tyramine-rich foods or sympathomimetics.
  - Foods with tyramine (red wine, cheese, chicken liver, fava beans, cured meats) cause a buildup of stored catecholamines.
  - In addition to a markedly elevated BP, it is also characterized by headache, sweating, nausea and vomiting, photophobia, autonomic instability, chest pain, arrhythmias, and death.
- Orthostatic hypotension (most common).
- Drowsiness.

WARDS TIP

MAOIs are considered more effective than TCAs in depression with atypical features, characterized by hypersomnia, increased appetite, heavy feeling in extremities, and increased sensitivity to interpersonal rejection.

WARDS TIP

Selegiline (Emsam transdermal patch) is a MAOI used to treat depression that does not require following the dietary restrictions when used in low dosages. However, decongestants, opiates (such as meperidine, fentanyl, and tramadol), and serotonergic drugs must still be avoided.

WARDS TIP

First step when suspecting serotonin syndrome: Discontinue the medication(s). Next, provide supportive care and benzodiazepines. The serotonin antagonist cyproheptadine can also be used.

WARDS TIP

Warning about atypical antipsychotics: Although they are used to treat the behavioral symptoms of neurocognitive disorders (dementias) and delirium, studies show an increased risk of all-cause mortality and stroke when using these agents in the elderly.

- Weight gain.
- Sexual dysfunction.
- Dry mouth.
- Sleep dysfunction.
- Patients with pyridoxine deficiency can have numbness or paresthesias, so they should supplement with B_6.
- Liver toxicity, seizures, and edema (rare).
- *"Start low and go slow"* (low doses that are increased slowly).

Antidepressant Use in Other Disorders

- OCD: SSRIs (in high doses), TCAs (clomipramine).
- Panic disorder: SSRIs, SNRIs, TCAs, MAOIs.
- Eating disorders: SSRIs (in high doses), TCAs.
- Persistent depressive disorder (dysthymia): SSRIs, SNRIs (e.g., venlafaxine, duloxetine).
- Social anxiety disorder (social phobia): SSRIs, SNRIs, MAOIs.
- GAD: SSRIs, SNRIs (venlafaxine), TCAs.
- Posttraumatic stress disorder: SSRIs.
- Irritable bowel syndrome: SSRIs, TCAs.
- Enuresis: TCAs (imipramine).
- Neuropathic pain: TCAs (amitriptyline and nortriptyline), SNRIs.
- Chronic pain: SNRIs, TCAs.
- Fibromyalgia: SNRIs.
- Migraine headaches: TCAs (amitriptyline).
- Smoking cessation: Bupropion.
- Premenstrual dysphoric disorder: SSRIs.
- Insomnia: Mirtazapine, trazodone, TCAs (doxepin).

Antipsychotics

- Antipsychotics are used to treat psychotic disorders as well as psychotic symptoms associated with other psychiatric and medical illnesses.
    - *Typical* or *first-generation* antipsychotics, sometimes referred to as neuroleptics, are classified according to potency and treat psychosis by blocking dopamine (D2) receptors.
    - *Atypical* or *second-generation* antipsychotics block both dopamine (D2) and serotonin (2A) receptors.
- Most antipsychotics have a number of actions and receptor interactions in the brain that contribute to their varied efficacy and side-effect profiles.
- Both typical and atypical antipsychotics have similar efficacies in treating the presence of *positive psychotic symptoms*, such as hallucinations and delusions.
- Atypical antipsychotics were thought to be more effective at treating *negative symptoms* (such as flattened affect and social withdrawal), although this has not been consistently shown in the literature.
- Atypical antipsychotics have largely replaced typical antipsychotics in use due to their favorable side-effect profile. However, the risk of metabolic syndrome/weight gain and other side effects, as well as the significant cost of the atypical antipsychotics means that currently both classes are used as first-line treatments.
- The choice of which specific medication to prescribe should be made based on the patient's individual clinical presentation, past response (favorable and unfavorable), side-effect profile, and preference.

TYPICAL (FIRST-GENERATION) ANTIPSYCHOTICS

All typical antipsychotics have similar efficacy, but vary in potency.

Low-Potency, Typical Antipsychotics
- Lower affinity for dopamine receptors and therefore a higher dose is required. Remember, *potency* refers to the action on dopamine receptors, *not* the level of efficacy.
- Higher incidence of antiadrenergic, anticholinergic, and antihistaminic side effects compared to high-potency typical antipsychotics.
- Lower incidence of EPS and (possibly) neuroleptic malignant syndrome.
- More lethality in overdose due to QTc prolongation, and the potential for heart block and ventricular tachycardia.
- Rare risk for agranulocytosis, and slightly higher seizure risk than high-potency antipsychotics.
  - **Chlorpromazine (Thorazine):**
    - Commonly causes orthostatic hypotension.
    - Can cause blue-gray skin discoloration as well as corneal and lens deposits.
    - Can lead to photosensitivity.
    - Also used to treat nausea and vomiting, as well as intractable hiccups.
  - **Thioridazine (Mellaril):** Associated with retinitis pigmentosa.

Midpotency, Typical Antipsychotics
- Have midrange properties.
  - **Loxapine (Loxitane):**
    - Higher risk of seizures.
    - Metabolite is an antidepressant.
  - **Thiothixene (Navane):** Can cause ocular pigment changes.
  - **Molindone (Moban).**
  - **Perphenazine (Trilafon).**

High-Potency, Typical Antipsychotics
- Greater affinity for dopamine receptors; therefore, a relatively low dose is needed to achieve effect.
- Less sedation, orthostatic hypotension, and anticholinergic effects.
- Greater risk for extrapyramidal symptoms and (likely) TD.
  - **Haloperidol (Haldol):** Can be given PO/IM/IV. Decanoate (long acting) form available.
  - **Fluphenazine (Prolixin):** Decanoate form available.
  - **Trifluoperazine (Stelazine):** Approved for nonpsychotic anxiety.
  - **Pimozide (Orap):** Associated with QTc prolongation and ventricular tachycardia.

Ms. Brown is a 28-year-old, overweight woman who presents to your outpatient clinic following discharge from an inpatient psychiatry unit. Police found her in a local shopping mall, talking to herself and telling a passersby that the devil had "stolen her soul." She appeared disheveled and scared. During the hospitalization, she was diagnosed with schizophrenia, and olanzapine was prescribed and titrated to 30 mg at bedtime for delusional thinking and disorganized behavior. She has since been living with her parents, and her hygiene and self-care have improved. Although Ms. Brown reports occasional auditory hallucinations telling her that her parents do not like her, she recognizes that the voices are not real and is not distressed by them. Ms. Brown has become involved in a vocational skills program and hopes to work at a local supermarket. However, during her last appointment with her primary care doctor, she was told she had an elevated fasting glucose of 115 and triglycerides of 180, and that she had gained 12 pounds in the past 3 months with a waist circumference of 36 inches. Her blood pressure was normal, but she reported a family history of diabetes and high blood pressure.

What is the next step?

Given her diagnosis of schizophrenia, and that Ms. Brown has had an adequate partial response to pharmacological treatment, she should continue to be treated with an antipsychotic. However, her recent laboratory results are suggestive of metabolic syndrome, and thus she is at an increased risk for cardiovascular disease. While this patient has responded well to olanzapine, this medication along with other atypical antipsychotics have been associated with increased weight gain and impaired glucose metabolism. It is unclear if Ms. Brown's laboratory test results were abnormal prior to starting olanzapine, are elevated secondary to treatment, or a combination of both. In treating Ms. Brown, first steps include recommending lifestyle modifications and close monitoring of her weight, blood sugar levels, lipids, and waist circumference, while collaborating closely with her primary care physician. If a change in her antipsychotic medication is warranted after weighing the risks and benefits of altering her treatment, other atypical antipsychotics such as ziprasidone or aripiprazole (both less associated with weight gain), or typical antipsychotics might be considered; these medications would then be cross-tapered. When choosing medications, consideration must be given to a history of response, tolerability, side-effect profile, patient preference, and cost.

KEY FACT

Haloperidol (Haldol) is often given as an intramuscular injection to treat acute agitation or psychosis.

WARDS TIP

Haloperidol and fluphenazine are also available in long-acting, intramuscular forms (decanoate) that are useful if patients are poorly compliant with their oral medication. Risperidone (Consta), aripiprazole (Maintena), and paliperidone (Invega Sustenna) also have long-acting injectables, but they are more expensive.

Side Effects

- The positive symptoms of schizophrenia are treated by action of the medications in the mesolimbic dopamine pathway. The mesolimbic pathway includes the nucleus accumbens, the fornix, the amygdala, and the hippocampus.
- The negative symptoms of schizophrenia are thought to occur due to (decreased) dopaminergic action in the mesocortical pathway.
- Extrapyramidal symptoms occur through blockade of the dopamine pathways in the nigrostriatum.
- Increased prolactin is caused by dopamine blockade in the tuberoinfundibular area.
- **Antidopaminergic effects:**
    - EPS:
        - *Parkinsonism*—bradykinesia, masklike face, cogwheel rigidity, pill-rolling tremor.
        - *Akathisia*—subjective anxiety and restlessness, objective fidgetiness. Patients may report a sensation of inability to sit still. Best treated with β-blockers or benzodiazepines.
        - *Dystonia*—sustained painful contraction of muscles of neck *(torticollis)*, tongue, eyes *(oculogyric crisis)*. It can be life threatening if it involves the airway or diaphragm.
    - **Hyperprolactinemia**—Leads to decreased libido, galactorrhea, gynecomastia, impotence, amenorrhea.

- **Anti-HAM effects:** Caused by actions on **H**istaminic, **A**drenergic, and **M**uscarinic receptors:
    - *Antihistaminic*—results in sedation, **weight gain**.
    - *Anti-α1 adrenergic*—results in orthostatic hypotension, cardiac abnormalities, and sexual dysfunction.
    - *Antimuscarinic*—anticholinergic effects, resulting in dry mouth, tachycardia, urinary retention, blurry vision, constipation, and precipitation of narrow-angle glaucoma.
- **Tardive dyskinesia:**
    - Choreoathetoid (writhing) movements of mouth and tongue (or other body parts) that may occur in patients who have used neuroleptics for more than 6 months.
    - Older age is a risk factor.
    - Women and patients with affective disorders *may* be at an increased risk.
    - Although 50% of cases will remit (without further antipsychotic use), most cases are *permanent*.
    - Treatment involves discontinuation of current antipsychotic if clinically possible and changing to a medication with less potential to cause TD.
- Less common side effects include **neuroleptic malignant syndrome:**
    - Though rare, occurs more often in *young males early in treatment* with *high-potency typical antipsychotics*.
    - It is a **medical emergency** and has up to a 20% mortality rate if left untreated.
    - It is characterized by:
        - **F**ever (most common presenting symptom).
        - **A**utonomic instability (tachycardia, labile hypertension, diaphoresis).
        - **L**eukocytosis.
        - **T**remor.
        - **E**levated CPK.
        - **R**igidity (*lead pipe* rigidity is considered almost universal).
        - **E**xcessive sweating (diaphoresis).
        - **D**elirium (mental status changes).
    - **Treatment** involves discontinuation of current medications and administration of supportive medical care (hydration, cooling, etc.).
    - Sodium dantrolene, bromocriptine, and amantadine may be used but have their own side effects and unclear efficacy.
    - This is *not* an allergic reaction.
    - Patient is not prevented from restarting the same neuroleptic at a later time, but will have an increased risk for another episode of neuroleptic malignant syndrome.
- Elevated liver enzymes, jaundice.
- **Ophthalmologic** problems (irreversible retinal pigmentation with high doses of thioridazine, deposits in lens and cornea with chlorpromazine).
- **Dermatologic** problems, including rashes and photosensitivity (blue-gray skin discoloration with chlorpromazine).
- **Seizures:** All antipsychotics lower the seizure threshold, although low-potency antipsychotics are more likely.

ATYPICAL (SECOND-GENERATION) ANTIPSYCHOTICS

- Atypical antipsychotics block both dopamine and serotonin receptors and are associated with different side effects than typical antipsychotics.
- In particular, they are less likely to cause EPS, TD, or neuroleptic malignant syndrome.

KEY FACT

There is a roughly 5% chance of developing tardive dyskinesia for each year treated with a typical antipsychotic.

KEY FACT

The first-line treatment for dystonia caused by antipsychotics is benztropine (Cogentin). Diphenhydramine (Benadryl) can also be used. The first-line treatment for akathisia is decreasing the dose of the causative agent (if appropriate). The second-line treatment is adding propranolol or a benzodiazepine.

KEY FACT

Clozapine, the first atypical antipsychotic, is less likely to cause tardive dyskinesia.

- They *may* be more effective in treating **negative symptoms** of schizophrenia than typical antipsychotics.
- Atypical antipsychotics are also used to treat acute mania, bipolar disorder, and as adjunctive medications in unipolar depression.
- They are also used in treating borderline personality disorder, PTSD, and certain psychiatric disorders in childhood (e.g., tic disorders).
  - **Clozapine (Clozaril):**
    - Less likely to cause tardive dyskinesia.
    - Only antipsychotic shown to be **more efficacious** than the others; used in **treatment refractory schizophrenia**.
    - Only antipsychotic shown to decrease **the risk of suicide**.
    - More anticholinergic side effects than other atypical or high-potency typical antipsychotics. Associated with tachycardia and hypersalivation.
    - **Risk of severe side effects**
      - One percent incidence of **agranulocytosis;** clozapine must be stopped if the *absolute neutrophil count* drops below 1500 per microliter.
      - Four percent incidence of **seizures**.
      - Small risk of **myocarditis**.
  - **Risperidone (Risperdal):**
    - Can cause increased prolactin.
    - Associated with orthostatic hypotension and reflex tachycardia.
    - Long-acting injectable form named Consta.
  - **Quetiapine (Seroquel):** Much less likely to cause EPS; common side effects include sedation and orthostatic hypotension.
  - **Olanzapine (Zyprexa):** Common side effects include weight gain, sedation, and dyslipidemia.
  - **Ziprasidone (Geodon):** Less likely to cause significant weight gain, associated with QTc prolongation, and must be taken with food (50% reduction in absorption without a 300-calorie meal).
  - **Aripiprazole (Abilify):**
    - Unique mechanism of partial D2 agonism.
    - Can be more activating (akathisia) and less sedating.
    - Less potential for weight gain.
- Newer (more expensive) antipsychotics:
  - **Paliperidone (Invega):**
    - Metabolite of risperidone.
    - Long-acting injectable form (Sustenna).
  - **Asenapine (Saphris) orally dissolving (sublingual) tablet.**
  - **Iloperidone (Fanapt).**
  - **Lurasidone (Latuda): Must be taken with food; used in bipolar depression.**

Side Effects

- **Metabolic syndrome.**
  - This must be monitored with baseline weight, waist circumference (measured at iliac crest), BP, HbA1c, and fasting lipids.
  - **Weight gain:** Metformin can be used to reduce or prevent.
  - Hyperlipidemia.
  - Hyperglycemia—rarely, **diabetic ketoacidosis** has been reported.
- Some anti-HAM effects (antihistaminic, antiadrenergic, and anti-muscarinic).
- Elevated liver function tests (LFTs)—monitor yearly for elevation in LFTs and ammonia.
- QTc prolongation.

Onset of Antipsychotic side effects

NMS: Any time (but usually early in treatment)
Acute dystonia: Hours to days
Parkinsonism/Akathisia: Days to weeks
Tardive dyskinesia: Months to years
The **Abnormal Involuntary Movement Scale (AIMS)** can be used to quantify and monitor for tardive dyskinesia.

Thirty percent of patients with treatment-resistant psychosis will respond to clozapine.

Patients on clozapine must have weekly blood draws for the first 6 months to check WBC and absolute neutrophil counts because of the risk of agranulocytosis. With time, the frequency of blood draws decreases.

Mood Stabilizers

- Mood stabilizers are used to treat **acute mania** and to help **prevent relapses** of manic episodes (maintenance treatment) in bipolar disorder and schizoaffective disorder. Less commonly, they may be used for:
  - Augmentation of antidepressants in patients with major depression refractory to monotherapy.
  - Potentiation of antipsychotics in patients with schizophrenia or schizoaffective disorder.
  - Treatment of aggression and impulsivity (e.g., neurocognitive disorders, intellectual disability, personality disorders, other medical conditions).
  - Enhancement of abstinence in treatment of alcoholism.
- Mood stabilizers include lithium and anticonvulsants, most commonly valproic acid, lamotrigine, and carbamazepine.

LITHIUM

- Lithium is the drug of choice in acute mania and as prophylaxis for both manic and depressive episodes in bipolar and schizoaffective disorders.
- It is also used in cyclothymic disorder and unipolar depression.
- Lithium is metabolized by the kidney, so dosing adjustments may be necessary in patients with renal dysfunction.
- Prior to initiating, patients should have an ECG, basic chemistries, thyroid function tests, a complete blood count (CBC), and a pregnancy test.
- Onset of action takes 5 to 7 days.
- Blood levels correlate with clinical efficacy and should be checked 4 to 5 days after every dose change.
- The major drawback of lithium is its high incidence of side effects and very narrow therapeutic index:
  - Therapeutic range: 0.6–1.2 (Individual patients can have significant side effects even within this range.)
  - Toxic: >1.5
  - Potentially lethal: >2.0

Side Effects

- Toxic levels of lithium cause altered mental status, coarse tremors, convulsions, delirium, coma, and death.
- Clinicians need to regularly monitor blood levels of lithium, thyroid function (thyroid-stimulating hormone), and kidney function.
- Fine tremor.
- Nephrogenic diabetes insipidus.
- GI disturbance.
- Weight gain.
- Sedation.
- Thyroid enlargement, hypothyroidism.
- ECG changes.
- Benign leukocytosis.
- Lithium may cause **Ebstein's anomaly**, a cardiac defect in babies born to mothers taking lithium.

WARDS TIP

Quetiapine, olanzapine, aripiprazole, risperidone, asenapine, and ziprasidone have FDA approval for treatment of mania.

WARDS TIP

Antipsychotics may be used as adjuncts to mood stabilizers early in the course of a manic episode. Atypical antipsychotics are often prescribed as monotherapy in the acute or maintenance treatment of bipolar disorder.

KEY FACT

Lithium is the only mood stabilizer shown to decrease suicidality.

KEY FACT

When prescribing lithium, it is important to monitor lithium levels, creatinine, and thyroid function tests.

WARDS TIP

Blood levels are useful for lithium, valproic acid, carbamazepine, and clozapine.

WARDS TIP

Be careful of prescribing ibuprofen or other nonsteroidal anti-inflammatory drugs (NSAIDs) to a patient on lithium.

WARDS TIP

Factors that increase Li+ levels:
- NSAIDs
- Aspirin (+/–)
- Thiazide diuretics
- Dehydration
- Salt deprivation
- Sweating (salt loss)
- Impaired renal function

WARDS TIP

Lithium's side effect of leukocytosis can be advantageous when combined with other medications that decrease WBC count (e.g., clozapine).

Anticonvulsants

CARBAMAZEPINE (TEGRETOL)

- Especially useful in treating mania with *mixed features* and *rapid-cycling* bipolar disorder; less effective for the depressed phase.
- Acts by blocking sodium channels and inhibiting action potentials.
- Onset of action is 5 to 7 days.
- Must check pregnancy test prior to initiating therapy as it increases the risk of neural tube defects.
- Carries risk of rash, SIADH, hyponatremia, benign leukopenia, and aplastic anemia (rare).
- CBC, LFTs must be obtained before initiating treatment and regularly monitored during treatment.
- Carbamazepine auto-induces its own metabolism. Patients may therefore need a dose increase in the first few weeks to months.
  - Serum carbamazepine levels should be measured initially and at 3, 6, and 9 weeks. Goal level is 4 to 12 mcg/mL.

Side Effects

- The most common side effects are GI and CNS (e.g., drowsiness, ataxia, sedation, confusion).
- Possible skin rash **(Stevens–Johnson syndrome)**.
- Leukopenia, hyponatremia, aplastic anemia, thrombocytopenia, and agranulocytosis.
- Elevation of liver enzymes, causing hepatitis.
- **Teratogenic** effects when used during pregnancy (neural tube defects).
- Significant drug interactions with many medications metabolized by the cytochrome P450 pathway, including inducing its own metabolism through *autoinduction* (requiring increasing dosages).
- Toxicity: Confusion, stupor, motor restlessness, ataxia, tremor, nystagmus, twitching, and vomiting.

VALPROIC ACID (DEPAKOTE AND DEPAKENE)

- Useful in treating acute mania, mania with mixed features, and rapid cycling.
- Multiple mechanisms of action: blocks sodium channels and increases GABA concentrations in the brain.
- Monitoring of LFTs and CBC is necessary.
- Drug levels should be checked after 4 to 5 days. Therapeutic range is 50–150 µg/mL.
- Contraindicated in pregnancy, so care should be given in women of childbearing age (neural tube defects).

Lamotrigine (Lamictal)
- Efficacy for **bipolar depression,** though little efficacy for acute mania or prevention of mania.
- Believed to work on sodium channels that modulate glutamate and aspartate.
- Most common side effects are dizziness, sedation, headaches, and ataxia.
- Most serious side effect is **Stevens–Johnson syndrome** (life-threatening rash involving skin and mucous membranes) in 0.1%. This is most likely in the first 2 to 8 weeks, but is minimized by starting with low doses and increasing *slowly*.

- Valproate will increase lamotrigine levels, and lamotrigine will decrease valproate levels.

Oxcarbazepine (Trileptal)
- As effective in mood disorders as carbamazepine, but better tolerated.
- Less risk of rash and hepatic toxicity.
- Monitor sodium levels for hyponatremia.

Gabapentin (Neurontin)
- Often used adjunctively to help with anxiety, sleep, neuropathic pain.
- Little efficacy in bipolar disorder.

Pregabalin (Lyrica)
- Used in GAD (second-line) and fibromyalgia.
- Little efficacy in bipolar disorder.

Tiagabine (Gabitril): Questionable benefit in treating anxiety

Topiramate (Topamax)
- May be helpful with impulse control disorders.
- Beneficial side effect is **weight loss.**
- Can cause hypochloremic, metabolic acidosis as well as kidney stones.
- The most limiting side effect is **cognitive slowing.**

Side Effects
- GI symptoms.
- Weight gain.
- Sedation.
- Alopecia.
- Pancreatitis.
- **Hepatotoxicity** or benign aminotransferase elevations.
- Increase in ammonia.
- Thrombocytopenia.
- **Teratogenic** effects during pregnancy (neural tube defects).

Anxiolytics/Hypnotics

- Include benzodiazepines (BDZs), barbiturates, and buspirone.
- Common indications for anxiolytics/hypnotics include:
    - Anxiety disorders.
    - Muscle spasm.
    - Seizures.
    - Sleep disorders.
    - Alcohol withdrawal.
    - Anesthesia induction.

WARDS TIP

BDZs can be lethal when mixed with alcohol. Respiratory depression may cause death.

BENZODIAZEPINES

- BDZs are the most widely prescribed psychotropic medications.
- BDZs work by potentiating the effects of gamma-aminobutyric acid (GABA).
- They reduce anxiety and can be used to treat akathisia.
- Many patients become physically dependent on these medications and require increasing amounts for the same clinical effect (i.e., tolerance).
- Potential for abuse.
- Choice of BDZ is based on time to onset of action, duration of action, and method of metabolism.

WARDS TIP

In chronic alcoholics or those with liver disease, use benzodiazepines that are not metabolized by the liver. There are a **LOT** of them:
Lorazepam
Oxazepam
Temazepam

- Relatively safer in overdose than barbiturates.
- **Long Acting (Half-life: >20 Hours)**
  - **Diazepam (Valium):**
    - Rapid onset.
    - Used during detoxification from alcohol or sedative-hypnotic-anxiolytics, and for seizures.
    - Effective for muscle spasm.
    - Less commonly prescribed to treat anxiety because of euphoria.
  - **Clonazepam (Klonopin):**
    - Treatment of anxiety, including panic attacks.
    - Avoid with renal dysfunction; longer half-life allows for once or twice daily dosing.
- **Intermediate Acting (Half-life: 6–20 Hours)**
  - **Alprazolam (Xanax):**
    - Treatment of anxiety, including panic attacks.
    - Short onset of action leads to euphoria, high abuse potential.
  - **Lorazepam (Ativan):**
    - Treatment of panic attacks, alcohol and sedative-hypnotic-anxiolytic detoxification, agitation.
    - Not metabolized by liver.
  - **Oxazepam (Serax):**
    - Alcohol and sedative-hypnotic-anxiolytic detoxification.
    - Not metabolized by liver.
  - **Temazepam (Restoril):**
    - Because of dependence, rarely used for treatment of insomnia.
    - Not metabolized by liver.
- **Short Acting (Half-life: <6 Hours)**
  - **Midazolam (Versed):**
    - **Very short half-life.**
    - Primarily used in medical and surgical settings.

WARDS TIP

For benzodiazepine overdose, flumazenil is used to reverse the effects. However, be careful not to induce withdrawal too quickly—this can be life threatening.

Side Effects

- Drowsiness.
- Impairment of intellectual function.
- Reduced motor coordination (careful in elderly).
- Anterograde amnesia.
- Withdrawal can be life threatening and cause seizures.
- Toxicity: Respiratory depression in overdose, especially when combined with alcohol.

NON-BDZ HYPNOTICS

- **Zolpidem (Ambien)/zaleplon (Sonata)/eszopiclone (Lunesta):**
  - Work by selective receptor binding to the omega-1 receptor on the GABA-A receptor, which is responsible for sedation.
  - Should be used for short-term treatment of insomnia.
  - Compared to BDZs, less tolerance/dependence occurs with prolonged use (but still can occur).
  - Zaleplon has a shorter half-life than zolpidem, which has a shorter half-life than eszopiclone.
  - Reports of anterograde amnesia, hallucinations, parasomnias (sleep-walking), and GI side effects may limit their tolerability.
- **Diphenhydramine (Benadryl):**
  - An antihistamine with moderate anticholinergic effects.
  - Side effects include sedation, dry mouth, constipation, urinary retention, and blurry vision.

- **Ramelteon (Rozerem):**
  - Selective melatonin MT_1 and MT_2 agonist.
  - No tolerance or dependence.

NON-BDZ ANXIOLYTICS

- **Buspirone (BuSpar):**
  - Partial agonist at 5HT-1A receptor, thereby decreasing serotonergic activity.
  - Slower onset of action than BDZs (takes several weeks for effect).
  - Not considered as effective as other options, and so it is often used in combination with another agent (e.g., an SSRI) for the treatment of generalized anxiety disorder.
  - Does not potentiate the CNS depression of alcohol (useful in alcoholics), and has a low potential for abuse/addiction.
- **Hydroxyzine (Atarax):**
  - An antihistamine.
  - Side effects include sedation, dry mouth, constipation, urinary retention, and blurry vision.
  - Useful for patients who want quick-acting, short-term medication, but who cannot take BDZs for various reasons.
- **Barbiturates** (e.g., **butalbitol, phenobarbital, amobarbitol, pentobarbital**): Rarely used because of the lethality of overdose, potential for abuse, and side-effect profile.
- **Propranolol:**
  - Beta-blocker.
  - Useful in treating the autonomic effects of panic attacks or social phobia (i.e., performance anxiety), such as palpitations, sweating, and tachycardia.
  - It can also be used to treat akathisia (side effect of antipsychotics).

Psychostimulants

Used in ADHD and in treatment refractory depression.
- **Dextroamphetamine and amphetamines (Dexedrine, Adderall):**
  - Dextroamphetamine is the D-isomer of amphetamine.
  - Schedule II due to high potential for **abuse/diversion.**
  - Monitor BP, and watch for weight loss, insomnia, exacerbation of tics, decreased seizure threshold.
- **Methylphenidate (Ritalin, Concerta):**
  - CNS stimulant, similar to amphetamine.
  - Schedule II.
  - Watch for leukopenia or anemia.
  - Monitor BP and CBC with differential, and watch for weight loss, insomnia, exacerbation of tics, decreased seizure threshold.
- **Atomoxetine (Strattera):**
  - Inhibits presynaptic norepinephrine reuptake, resulting in increased synaptic norepinephrine and dopamine.
  - Less appetite suppression and insomnia.
  - Not classified as a controlled substance.
  - Less abuse potential than dextroamphetamine/methylphenidate but less effective.
  - Rare liver toxicity, and possible increase in suicidal ideation in children/adolescents.
- **Modafinil (Provigil):** Used in narcolepsy, not ADHD.

Cognitive Enhancers

Used in major neurocognitive disorders (dementias).

ACETYLCHOLINESTERASE INHIBITORS

- **Donepezil (Aricept):**
    - Once-daily dosing.
    - Some GI side effects.
    - Used in mild-to-moderate neurocognitive disorders (dementias).
- **Galantamine (Razadyne):**
    - Twice-daily dosing.
    - GI side effects.
    - Used in mild-to-moderate neurocognitive disorders (dementias).
- **Rivastigmine (Exelon):**
    - Twice-daily dosing.
    - Has daily patch form, with fewer side effects.
    - Used in mild-to-moderate neurocognitive disorders (dementias).

NMDA (GLUTAMATE) RECEPTOR ANTAGONIST

- **Memantine (Namenda):**
    - Used in moderate-to-severe neurocognitive disorders (dementia).
    - Fewer side effects than cholinesterase inhibitors.
    - Should be used in conjunction with acetylcholinesterase inhibitor.

> **KEY FACT**
>
> Alzheimer's medications, such as donepezil and rivastigmine, work by reversible inhibition of acetylcholine esterase.

Reference List of Medications That May Cause Psychiatric Symptoms

PSYCHOSIS

Sympathomimetics, analgesics, antibiotics (e.g., isoniazid, antimalarials), anticholinergics, anticonvulsants, antihistamines, corticosteroids, antiparkinsonian agents.

AGITATION/CONFUSION/DELIRIUM

Antipsychotics, **anticholinergics**, **antihistamines**, antidepressants, antiarrhythmics, antineoplastics, corticosteroids, NSAIDs, antiasthmatics, antibiotics, antihypertensives, antiparkinsonian agents, thyroid hormones.

DEPRESSION

Antihypertensives, antiparkinsonian agents, **corticosteroids**, calcium channel blockers, NSAIDs, antibiotics, peptic ulcer drugs.

ANXIETY

Sympathomimetics, antiasthmatics, antiparkinsonian agents, hypoglycemic agents, NSAIDs, thyroid hormones.

SEDATION/POOR CONCENTRATION

Antianxiety agents/hypnotics, anticholinergics, mood stabilizers, antibiotics, antihistamines, antipsychotics (e.g., clozapine, quetiapine, olanzapine).

SELECTED MEDICATIONS

- **Procainamide, quinidine:** Confusion, delirium.
- **Albuterol:** Anxiety, confusion.
- **Isoniazid:** Psychosis.
- **Tetracycline:** Depression.
- **Nifedipine, verapamil:** Depression.
- **Cimetidine:** Depression, confusion, psychosis.
- **Steroids:** Aggressiveness/agitation, mania, depression, anxiety, psychosis.

Other Treatments

ELECTROCONVULSIVE THERAPY (ECT)

Patients are often premedicated with atropine, and then given general anesthesia (typically with methohexital) and muscle relaxants (e.g., succinylcholine). A generalized tonic-clonic seizure is then induced using unilateral or bilateral electrodes. While the mechanism of action of ECT is not fully known, there are likely anticonvulsant effects, as well as brain perfusion and connectivity changes involved. ECT is **the most effective** treatment for major depressive disorder, especially with psychotic features, as well as for acute mania and catatonia. It is often used in patients who cannot tolerate medications or who have failed other treatments. ECT is discontinued after symptomatic improvement, typically a course of 8 to 12 sessions given three times weekly. Monthly *maintenance ECT* is often used to prevent relapse of symptoms. The most common side effects are muscle soreness, headaches, amnesia, and confusion. Bilateral electrode placement is more efficacious, but increases memory impairment and confusion.

DEEP BRAIN STIMULATION (DBS)

DBS is a surgical treatment involving the implantation of a medical device that sends electrical impulses to specific parts of the brain. DBS in select brain regions has provided benefits for Parkinson disease and disabling dystonia, as well as for chronic pain and tremors. Its underlying principles and mechanisms are still not clear. DBS directly changes brain activity in a controlled manner and its effects are reversible (unlike those of lesioning techniques). DBS has been used to treat various affective disorders, including major depression. While DBS has proven helpful for some patients, there is potential for serious complications and side effects.

REPETITIVE TRANSCRANIAL MAGNETIC STIMULATION (rTMS)

rTMS is a noninvasive method to excite neurons in the brain. Weak electric currents are induced in the tissue by rapidly changing magnetic fields, a process called electromagnetic induction. In this way, brain activity can be triggered with minimal discomfort. rTMS can produce longer-lasting changes than nonrepetitive stimulation. Numerous small-scale studies have demonstrated efficacy in the treatment of major depression; however, studies show less efficacy than for ECT, and the price of treatment is high. Side effects include seizures (rare), as well as headache and scalp pain.

LIGHT THERAPY

Light therapy, or phototherapy, consists of exposure to daylight or to specific wavelengths of light using lasers, light-emitting diodes, fluorescent lamps, dichroic lamps or very bright, full-spectrum light, for a prescribed amount of time and, in some cases, at a specific time of day. Light therapy is used to treat major depression with a seasonal pattern (**seasonal affective disorder**), with some support for its use with nonseasonal psychiatric disorders.

KETAMINE INFUSION

Ketamine is a NMDA receptor antagonist that is most commonly used as an anesthetic agent. Ketamine can be given as an IV infusion for the treatment of unipolar major depression. It's effect is rapid (with response within 40 to 120 minutes), but the effect dissipates by day 10 to 14. Ketamine carries a risk of dissociation/psychosis, bladder toxicity, and neurotoxicity. Currently, use of IV ketamine for depression is largely limited to research settings.

CHAPTER 19

FORENSIC PSYCHIATRY

Standard of Care and Malpractice	212	Competence to Stand Trial	215
Confidentiality	212	Not Guilty by Reason of Insanity (NGRI)	216
Decision Making	213	Risk Assessment	216
EMANCIPATED MINORS	213	Malingering	217
DECISIONAL CAPACITY	214	Child and Family Law	217
GUARDIANS AND CONSERVATORS	215	Correctional Psychiatry	217
Admission to a Psychiatric Hospital	215		
Disability	215		

Forensic psychiatry is a medical subspecialty that includes areas in which psychiatry is applied to legal matters. Forensic psychiatrists often conduct evaluations requested by the court or attorneys.

While some (forensic) psychiatrists specialize exclusively in legal issues, almost all psychiatrists have to work within one of the many spheres where the mental health and legal system overlap. These areas include the following:

- Risk assessment.
- Criminal responsibility.
- Competence/decisional capacity.
- Child custody and visitation.
- Psychic trauma.
- Mental disability.
- Malpractice.
- Involuntary treatment.
- Correctional psychiatry.

Legal issues are considered **criminal** in nature if someone is being charged with a crime. **Civil** cases involve other kinds of rights and may result in monetary awards. It is important to note that the specific laws pertaining to the various topics discussed in this chapter may vary by state.

WARDS TIP

A wrong prediction or a bad outcome is not necessarily proof of bad doctoring (malpractice).

Standard of Care and Malpractice

- The **standard of care** in psychiatry is generally defined as the skill level and knowledge base of the average, prudent psychiatrist in a given community.
- **Negligence** is practicing below the standard of care.
- **Malpractice** is the act of being negligent as a doctor.
- The following four conditions typically must be proven by a preponderance of the evidence in order to sustain a claim of malpractice:
    1. The physician had a duty of care (psychiatrist–patient relationship).
    2. The physician breached his or her duty by practice that did not meet the standard of care (negligence).
    3. The patient was harmed.
    4. The harm was directly caused by the physician's negligence.
- If a malpractice case is successful, the patient can receive **compensatory damages** (reimbursement for medical expenses, lost salary, or physical suffering) and **punitive damages** (money awarded to "punish" the doctor).

KEY FACT

Four Ds of malpractice: Deviation (neglect) from Duty that was the Direct cause of Damage.

KEY FACT

The obligation of a physician to report patients who are potentially dangerous to others is called the *Tarasoff duty* or *duty to warn*, which was based on a landmark legal case.

Confidentiality

All information regarding a doctor–patient relationship should be held confidential, except when otherwise exempted by statute, such as:

- When sharing relevant information with other staff members who are also treating the patient.
- If subpoenaed—physician must supply all requested information.
- If child abuse is suspected—obligated to report to the proper authorities.
- If a patient is suicidal—physician may need to admit the patient, with or without the patient's consent, and share information with the hospital staff.
- If a patient threatens direct harm to another person—physician may have a duty to warn the intended victim.

KEY FACT

Doctors are required to report child abuse, but lawyers are not.

Decision Making

- Process by which patients knowingly and voluntarily agree to a treatment or procedure.
- In order to make informed decisions, patients must know the purpose of the treatment, alternative treatments, and the potential risks and benefits of undergoing and of refusing the treatment.
- The patient should have the opportunity to ask questions.
- Situations that do not require informed consent:
    - Lifesaving medical emergency.
    - Prevention of suicidal or homicidal behavior.
    - Unemancipated minors (typically require informed consent from the parent or legal guardian).

EMANCIPATED MINORS

- Considered competent to give consent for all medical care without parental input or consent.
- Minors are considered emancipated if they are:
    - Self-supporting.
    - In the military.
    - Married.
    - Have children **or pregnant.**

> **KEY FACT**
>
> Elements of informed consent (4 Rs):
> - **R**eason for treatment
> - **R**isks and benefits
> - **R**easonable alternatives
> - **R**efused treatment consequences

A 74-year-old African-American male with insulin-dependent diabetes mellitus and severe major depressive disorder was admitted to the intensive care unit for treatment of diabetic ketoacidosis. The internal medicine team calls your psychiatry consult-liaison service to evaluate the patient for depression and provide treatment recommendations.

When you meet the patient, he is disoriented, confused, and has a waxing and waning level of consciousness. His mini-mental state exam (MMSE) score is 18/30. You identify that the patient is likely delirious, and you are unable to obtain any useful historical information. After interviewing the patient's daughter by phone, you learn that the patient's wife passed away 2 years ago, and in the past he had told family members that he can no longer live without her. One year ago, his daughter found him in the garage taping a hose to his car's exhaust pipe. She said that he broke down crying and admitted that he was going to kill himself by carbon monoxide poisoning. His daughter has been very concerned because he refuses to check his glucose or take his insulin as recommended. She stated, "I think he was trying to kill himself by not taking care of his diabetes."

He is followed daily by your consult-liaison team, and his MMSE score improves to 28/30. On hospital day 5, the internal medicine team informs you that he has developed wet gangrene in his right lower extremity and will need to have a below-knee amputation as soon as possible. The team asks you to assess the patient's capacity to make medical decisions because he is adamantly refusing to consent to this procedure.

You meet with the patient to discuss his medical situation. He is alert, lucid, and fully oriented. His affect is euthymic and appropriate. He states, "My doctor told me that I had an ulcer on my foot from poorly controlled diabetes that has become severely infected. I was told that I need to have my right leg amputated very soon or else I could die from the infection." He maintains that he is not interested in the surgical procedure that has been recommended. He adds, "My daughter is begging me to have the surgery, but I'm already old and I don't want to have to use a prosthetic leg or a wheelchair. I do not think life would be worth living if I had this amputation." He denies suicidal thoughts and intent.

Does this patient with history of severe major depressive disorder demonstrate the capacity to refuse a potentially life-saving procedure?

Yes, he demonstrates the capacity to refuse the recommended amputation. Legal standards for decision-making capacity to consent or refuse medical treatment involve the following: the ability to communicate a choice, to understand the relevant information, to appreciate the medical consequences of the situation, and to reason about treatment choices. In this case, the patient demonstrated the ability to discuss all of these topics. Although he was cognitively impaired on admission, his delirium eventually cleared.

However, the case is complicated by the fact that the patient may be currently suffering from major depression. This should be further assessed. While a history of current major depression does not preclude having decisional capacity, the patient should be evaluated carefully to ensure that his refusal of treatment does not stem from intent to commit suicide. If it does, then his suicidal intent would be interfering with his ability to reason. Optimally, the consult-liaison team may recommend treating the depression and readdressing the surgical procedure when his depression is in remission, but this may take many weeks and failure to amputate the limb in a timely manner could result in death. Since the patient demonstrates decision-making capacity and does not appear to be suicidal at this time, the medical team must respect the patient's wishes and treat the condition without surgery.

DECISIONAL CAPACITY

Competence and *capacity* are terms that refer to a patient's ability to make informed treatment decisions.

- *Capacity* is a clinical term and may be assessed by physicians.
- *Competence* is a legal term and can be decided only by a judge.
- Decisional capacity is *task specific* and can fluctuate over time.
- In order for a patient to have decisional capacity, he or she must be able to:
    - Understand the relevant information regarding treatment (purpose, risks, benefits).
    - Appreciate the appropriate weight and impact of the decision.
    - Logically manipulate the information to make a decision.
    - Communicate a choice or preference.
- Criteria for determining capacity may be more stringent if the consequences of a patient's decision are very serious.
- If a patient is determined not to have decisional capacity, the decision is typically made by a surrogate decision maker, usually a power of attorney, spouse, or close family member.

GUARDIANS AND CONSERVATORS

- May be appointed by a judge to make treatment decisions for incompetent patients.
- Make decisions by "substituted judgment." This means making decisions based on what the patient would most likely have wanted, were the patient competent.
- Patients can often express their wishes for treatment in advance of losing competence or capacity using a mental health advance directive form called "Declaration for Mental Health Treatment."

Admission to a Psychiatric Hospital

The two main categories of admission to a psychiatric hospital are voluntary and involuntary.

- **Voluntary:**
    - Patient requests or agrees to be admitted to the psychiatric ward.
    - Voluntary patients often have to meet the same symptom severity criteria as involuntary patients as listed below.
    - Voluntary patients may not have the right to be discharged immediately upon request.
    - Patient must have capacity and be competent to be admitted as a voluntary patient to an inpatient facility.
- **Involuntary:**
    - Patient must be found to be imminently at risk of harm to one's self or others or unable to provide for his/her basic needs.
    - Involuntary patients have legal rights to a trial to challenge their hospitalization.
    - Involuntary patients do not automatically lose the right to refuse treatment, including the involuntary administration of non-emergent medication.
    - Involuntary commitment is supported by legal principles of **police power** (protecting citizens from each other) and **parens patriae** (protecting citizens who can't care for themselves).

Disability

- **Mental impairment:** Any mental or psychological disorder.
- **Mental disability:** Alteration of an individual's capacity to meet personal, social, or occupational demands due to a mental impairment.
- To assess whether an impairment is also a disability, consider four categories:
    - Activities of daily living.
    - Social functioning.
    - Concentration, persistence, and pace.
    - Deterioration or decompensation in work settings.

Competence to Stand Trial

- *Competence* is a legal term for the capacity to understand, rationally manipulate, and apply information to make a reasoned decision on a specific issue. This definition varies by state.

> **KEY FACT**
>
> Emancipated minors do not need parental consent to make medical decisions.

> **WARDS TIP**
>
> If a child presents to the emergency department with various bruises, suspicious injuries in various stages of healing, and numerous prior emergency room visits, your next step would most likely be to contact the appropriate authorities.

> **KEY FACT**
>
> Sixth Amendment: Right to counsel, a speedy trial, and to confront witnesses

> **KEY FACT**
>
> Fourteenth Amendment: Right to due process of law

- The Sixth and Fourteenth Amendments to the Constitution are the basis for the law that someone cannot be tried if they are not mentally competent to stand trial.
- This was established by the legal case *Dusky v. United States* in 1960.
- If a defendant has significant mental health problems or behaves irrationally in court, his competency to stand trial should be considered.
- Competence to stand trial may change over time.
- To stand trial, a defendant must:
  - Understand the charges against him or her.
  - Be familiar with the courtroom personnel and procedure.
  - Have the ability to work with an attorney and participate in his or her trial.
  - Understand possible consequences.

KEY FACT

The fact that someone is mentally ill doesn't mean they aren't competent to stand trial.

Not Guilty by Reason of Insanity (NGRI)

- Conviction of a crime requires both an "evil deed" (*actus reus*) and "evil intent" (*mens rea*).
- **Insanity** is a legal term, and its definition varies by state (see Table 19-1).
- If someone is declared legally insane, they are not criminally responsible for their act.
- Some states have a ruling of Guilty but Mentally Ill (GBMI) instead of NGRI, or no criminal insanity defense at all.
- NGRI is used in less than 1% of criminal cases.
- It is successful in 26% of cases that continue to use it throughout the trial.
- Those found NGRI often spend the same amount of time (or more) as involuntary psychiatric patients than they would have spent in prison if they were found guilty.

WARDS TIP

After John Hinckley received NGRI for an assassination attempt on President Reagan, there was public outcry against lenient NGRI standards, contributing to the Insanity Defense Reform Act of 1984.

Risk Assessment

- Mental disorders are neither necessary nor sufficient causes of violence.
  - The major risk factors of violence are a history of violence, being young, male, and of lower socioeconomic status.
  - Substance use is a major determinant of violence, whether it occurs in the context of a mental illness or not.

TABLE 19-1. Insanity Defense Standards

Standard	Definition
M'Naghten	- Person did not understand what he/she was doing *or* its wrongfulness. - Most stringent test.
American Law Institute (ALI) Model Penal Code	Person could neither appreciate the criminality of his/her conduct *nor* conform his conduct to the requirements of the law.
Irresistible Impulse	Person could not appreciate right from wrong *or* could not control actions.
Durham	- The person's criminal act has resulted from mental illness. - Most lenient test and is rarely used.

- **Predicting dangerousness:**
    - Short-term easier than long-term.
    - High false positives because of low base rates (most people are not violent).

Malingering

- Feigning or exaggerating symptoms for "secondary gain," including:
    - Financial gain (injury law suit).
    - Avoiding school, work, or other responsibilities.
    - Obtaining medications of abuse (opioids, benzodiazepines).
    - Avoiding legal consequences.
- Signs for detecting malingering:
    - Atypical presentation.
    - "Textbook" description of the illness.
    - History of working in the medical field.
    - Symptoms that are present only when the patient knows he/she is being observed.
    - History of substance use or antisocial personality disorder.
    - Reluctant to engage in invasive/in-depth testing or treatment.

The most important factor in assessing a patient's risk of violence is the individual's history of violence.

The contribution of people with mental illness to overall rates of violence is small. People with mental illness are more likely to be the *victims* of violence than the perpetrators.

Child and Family Law

Evaluations for which a child forensic psychiatrist may be needed include:

- Child custody.
- Termination of parental rights.
- Child abuse or neglect.

Correctional Psychiatry

- With the closing of state psychiatric hospitals (i.e., deinstitutionalization), many persons with mental illness have moved to correctional institutions.
- Psychiatrists who practice in jails and prisons must balance treating the inmates as their patients and maintaining safety in the institution.
- Issues of **confidentiality** and **violence** are key.

CHAPTER 19: FORENSIC PSYCHIATRY

NOTES

INDEX

A

Abilify (aripiprazole), 28, 200, 202
Abnormal Involuntary Movement
    Scale (AIMS), 202
Abreaction, 134
Abuse. *See* Child abuse; Elder abuse
Acting out, 184
Acute dystonia, 28
    pocket card, 9
Acute stress disorder, 61–62
AD (Alzheimer disease), 103–104
ADHD (attention deficit/hyperactivity
    disorder), 123–125
Adjustment disorders, 62
Admission to a psychiatric hospital, 215
Advanced sleep phase disorder, 169
Affect, 14
AFRAID acronym for symptoms of avoidant personality
    disorder, 73
Aging
    normal, 112
    sexual changes with, 174
Agitation, medications causing, 208
Agoraphobia, 53
AIMS (Abnormal Involuntary
    Movement Scale), 202
Akathisia, 27, 192
Akinesia, 14
Albuterol
    may cause anxiety, confusion, 209
Alcohol (EtOH), 82–87
    alcohol use disorder, 85–87
        screening for (AUDIT-C acronym), 85–86
    intoxication, 82–83
    most common drug of abuse by adolescents, 128
    withdrawal, 83–84
Alcoholic hallucinosis, 16
Alcoholic ketoacidosis, 84
Alogia, 24
Alprazolam (Xanax), 206
Altruism, 183
Alzheimer disease (AD), 103–104
Ambien (zolpidem), 206
American Psychiatric Association (APA), 19
Amitriptyline (Elavil), 196
Amok, 32
Amoxapine (Asendin), 196
Amphetamine (Adderall), 207
Amphetamines, 88
Anafranil (clomipramine), 196
Analytically oriented (psychodynamic) psychotherapy
    sexual dysfunctions and paraphilic disorders, 177
Anhedonia, 24, 39
Anorexia nervosa, 155–157
    binge-eating/purging type, 155
    versus major depressive disorder, 156
    restricting type, 155
antiasthmatics
    may cause anxiety, 208
Anticholinergics
    may cause agitation, 209
    may cause confusion, 209
    may cause delirium, 209
Anticonvulsants, 204
    carbamazepine (Tegretol), 204
    valproic acid (Depakote and Depakene), 204–205
Antidepressant medications, 40–41, 193–198
    heterocyclic antidepressants, 196
    miscellaneous antidepressants, 195–196
    monoamine oxidase inhibitors, 197–198
    monoamine oxidase inhibitors (MAOIs). *See* Monoamine
        oxidase inhibitors (MAOIs)
    novel agents, 40
    selective serotonin reuptake inhibitors
        (SSRIs). *See* Selective Serotonin reuptake
        inhibitors (SSRIs)
    serotonin-norepinephrine reuptake inhibitors
        (SNRIs), 40, 195
    tetracyclic antidepressants, 196–197
    tricyclic antidepressants (TCAs), 9, 40, 196
    use in other disorders, 198
Anti-Ham effects, 201
Antihistamines
    may cause agitation, 209
    may cause confusion, 209
    may cause delirium, 209
Antipsychotic medications, 198–202
    atypical (second-generation)
        antipsychotics, 201–202
    important side effects, 28–29
    typical (first-generation) antipsychotics, 199–201
Antisocial personality disorder, 69–70
Anxiety disorders, 50–57
    agoraphobia, 53
    caffeine can increase, 56
    exercise can reduce, 56
    generalized anxiety disorder (GAD), 56–57
    medical conditions that can cause, 51
    medications and substances that can
        cause, 50, 208
    overview, 50–51
    panic attacks, 52
    panic disorder, 52–53
    pharmacotherapy, 51
    psychotherapy, 51
    selective mutism, 54–55
    separation anxiety disorder, 55
    signs and symptoms, 50
    social anxiety disorder (social phobia), 54
    specific phobias, 53–54
    treatment guidelines, 51

Anxiolytics/hypnotics, 205–207
    benzodiazepines, 205–206
    non-BDZ anxiolytics, 207
    non-BDZ hypnotics, 206–207
Anxious distress, 44
APA (American Psychiatric Association), 19
Appearance/behavior, 14
Aricept (donepezil), 208
Aripiprazole (Abilify, Maintena), 28, 200, 202
ASD (autism spectrum disorder), 125–126
Asenapine (Saphris), 28
Asendin (Amoxapine), 196
Atarax (hydroxyzine), 207
Ativan (lorazepam), 206
Atomoxetine (Strattera), 207
Attention deficit/hyperactivity disorder (ADHD), 123–125
Atypical (second-generation) antipsychotics, 201–202
Auditory hallucinations, 22
Autism spectrum disorder (ASD), 125–126
Automatisms, 14
Aventyl (nortriptyline), 196
Aversion therapy, 186
Avoidant personality disorder, 73–74
Avolition, 24

B

Balint, Michael, 182
Barbiturates, 207
    withdrawal, deadliness of, 90
Bedside cognitive testing, 17
    Mini-Mental State Examination (MMSE), 17
    Montreal Cognitive Assessment (MOCA), 17–18
Bedside manner, 2–3
Bed-wetting, 129
Behavioral modification
    oppositional defiant disorder, 127
Behavioral therapy, 186
    conditioning, 186
    deconditioning, 186–187
    learning theory, 186
    in schizophrenia, 28
Behavior modification
    oppositional defiant disorder (ODD), 128
Benadryl (diphenhydramine), 206
Benzodiazepines, 205–206
    anxiety disorders, 51
Bereavement, 42, 115
Bereavement-associated depression, 115
Beta-blockers
    anxiety disorders, 51
    panic attacks, 52
    performance anxiety, 52
Binge-eating disorder, 157–159
Biofeedback, 186–187
Bipolar disorders
    bipolar I disorder, 42–43
    bipolar II disorder, 43–44
    specifiers for, 44
Blood-injury-injection-specific phobia, 54
Body dysmorphic disorder, 58
Borderline personality disorder (BPD), 30, 70–71
Bradykinesia, 14
Brain fag, 32
Brief dynamic psychotherapy, 185
Brief psychotic disorder, 26, 30
    time course, 32
Bulimia nervosa, 157–158
    bupropion (Wellbutrin) could lower seizure threshold, 158
    dental caries and, 158
    fluoxetine is effective for, 158
Buprenorphine
    opioid use disorder, 91
Bupropion (Wellbutrin), 40, 195
Buspirone (BuSpar), 207
    anxiety disorders, 51

C

Caffeine, 94
    overdose, 94
    withdrawal, 94
CAM (Confusion Assessment Method), 100
Cannabis
    second most common drug of abuse by adolescents, 128
Capacity, 214
CAPRI mnemonic for personality disorders, 64
Carbamazepine (Tegretol), 204
Catatonia, 24, 42, 44
CBT (cognitive-behavioral therapy). *See* Cognitive-behavioral therapy (CBT)
Celexa (citalopram), 194
Central sleep apnea, 165–166
CHASES acronym for dysthymia, 45
Child abuse, 130–131
    doctors are mandated reporters, 130
    neglect, 131
    physical abuse, 130
        red flags for, 130
    psychological abuse, 130
    sequelae, 131
    sexual abuse
        red flags for, 130
        taking seriously, 130
    treatment, 131
Child and family law, 217
Children, psychiatric disorders in, 119–131
    attention deficit/hyperactivity disorder (ADHD), 123–125
    autism spectrum disorder (ASD), 125–126
    child abuse, 130–131
        neglect, 131
        physical abuse, 130
        psychological abuse, 130
        sequelae, 131
        sexual abuse, 130
        treatment, 131
    communication disorders, 122–123
    disruptive and conduct disorders, 127–128
        conduct disorder, 128
        oppositional defiant disorder (ODD), 127–128

elimination disorders, 129–130
global developmental delay, 121
  causes, 121
intellectual disability, 120–121
psychiatric examination, 120
  methods of gathering information, 120
  safety assessment, 120
  sources of information, 120
specific learning disorder (LD), 122
tic disorders, 126–127
Chlorpromazine (Thorazine), 28, 199
Cholinesterase inhibitors
  for Alzheimer disease, 104
Chorea, 108
Cigarette smoking during pregnancy, 94
Cimetidine
  may cause depression, confusion, psychosis, 209
Circadian rhythm sleep-wake disorders, 168–169
Circumstantiality, 15
Citalopram (Celexa), 194
Civil cases, 212
Clang associations, 15
Classical conditioning, 186
Classroom observation, 120
Clerkship (shelf) exam, preparing for, 4–9
  eat light, balanced meals, 4
  pocket cards, 5–9
  study in a bright room, 4
  study with friends, 4
  take practice exams, 4
  use question banks, 4
Clinical Opioid Withdrawal Scale (COWS), 92
Clomipramine (Anafranil), 196
Clonazepam (Klonopin), 206
Clozapine (Clozaril), 28–29, 202
Cluster A personality disorders, 65–68
  paranoid personality disorder (PPD), 65
  schizoid personality disorder, 66–67
  schizotypal personality disorder, 67–68
Cluster B personality disorders, 68–73
  antisocial personality disorder, 69–70
  borderline personality disorder (BPD), 70–71
  histrionic personality disorder (HPD), 71–72
  narcissistic personality disorder (NPD), 72–73
Cluster C personality disorders, 73–76
  avoidant personality disorder, 73–74
  dependent personality disorder (DPD), 74–75
  obsessive-compulsive personality disorder (OCPD), 75–76
  other specified personality disorder, 76
  personality change due to another medical condition, 76
  unspecified personality disorder, 76
Cocaine, 87–88
  cocaine use disorder, 87
  intoxication, 87
  withdrawal, 88
Cognition, 16
Cognitive-behavioral therapy (CBT), 187
  anxiety disorders, 51
  chronic insomnia, 163
  major depressive disorder, 41
  sexual dysfunctions and paraphilic disorders, 177

Cognitive enhancers, 208
  acetylcholinesterase inhibitors, 208
  NMDA (glutamate) receptor antagonist, 208
Cognitive processing therapy, 62
Cognitive symptoms of schizophrenia, 24
Cognitive therapy, 187
Collaborative couples therapy, 189
Command hallucinations, 22
Communication disorders in children, 122–123
Compensatory damages, 212
Competence, 214–216
Compulsions, 57
  common patterns, 57
Concerta (methylphenidate), 207
Concurrent couples therapy
Conditioning, 186
Conduct disorder, 69, 128
  cruelty to animals may be indicative, 128
  male versus female misconduct, 128
Confabulation, 84, 112
Confidentiality, 212, 217
Confusion, medications causing, 208
Confusion Assessment Method (CAM), 100
Conjoint couples therapy, 189
Conjunctival injection (red eyes), 93
Consta (risperidone), 28, 200
Constricted pupils, 90–91
Control, delusions of, 22
Controlling, 183
Conversion disorder (functional neurological symptom disorder), 141–142
Coprolalia, 126
Correctional psychiatry, 217
CORRUPT acronym for symptoms of antisocial personality disorder, 70
Countertransference, 185
Couples therapy, 189
  major depressive disorder, 41
COWS (Clinical Opioid Withdrawal Scale), 92
Creutzfeldt–Jakob disease, 109
Criminal cases, 212
Cruelty to animals
  may be indicative of conduct disorder, 128
Culture-specific psychoses, 32
Cyclothymic disorder, 45–46
Cymbalta (duloxetine), 40, 195

D

Date-rape drug (gamma-hydroxybutyrate), 89
DBT (dialectical behavior therapy), 71, 188
Decision making, 213–215
  decisional capacity, 214
  emancipated minors, 213
  guardians and conservators, 215
Deconditioning, 186–187
Deep brain stimulation (DBS), 209
Defense mechanisms, 182–184
  immature defenses, 184
  mature defenses, 183
  neurotic defenses, 183–184

Delayed ejaculation, 176
Delayed sleep phase disorder (DPSD), 169
Delirium, 98–100
    clinical manifestations, 99
    diagnosis, 100
    DSM-5 criteria, 100
    epidemiology, 98
    etiology, 98
    medical emergency, 98
    medications causing, 99, 208
    pocket card, 5–6
    precipitating factors, 98
    risk factors, 98
    treatment, 100–101
Delirium tremens (DTs)
    pocket card, 9
Delusional disorder, 31
    versus schizophrenia, 31
Delusional patients, interviewing, 18
Delusions, 15, 22
    classified by theme, 22, 31
        delusions of control, 22
        delusions of grandeur, 22
        delusions of guilt, 22
        delusions of persecution/paranoid delusions, 22
        erotomanic type, 31
        grandiose type, 31
        ideas of reference, 22
        jealous type, 31
        mixed type, 31
        persecutory type, 31
        somatic, 22, 31
        unspecified type, 31
    definition of, 22
    difference from illusions and hallucinations, 23
Denial, 184
Depakene (valproic acid), 204–205
Depakote (valproic acid), 204–205
Dependent personality disorder (DPD), 74–75
Depersonalization/derealization disorder, 135
Depressed patients, interviewing, 19
Depression
    major depression. *See* Major depressive disorder (MDD); Major depressive episode (MDE)
    medications causing, 208
    specifiers for, 41–42
Derealization, 135
Desipramine (Norpramin), 196
Desvenlafaxine (Pristiq), 195
Desyrel (trazodone), 195–196
    causes priapism, 195–196
Detection of substance use disorders, 81
Dextroamphetamine (Dexedrine), 207
Diagnosis. *See* Examination and diagnosis
Dialectical behavior therapy (DBT), 71, 188
Diazepam (Valium), 206
DIG FAST (mania), 37
    pocket card, 7
Diphenhydramine (Benadryl), 206
Disability, 215
Displacement, 183

Disruptive and conduct disorders, 127–128
    conduct disorder, 128
    oppositional defiant disorder (ODD), 127–128
Disruptive mood dysregulation disorder (DMDD), 46–47
Dissociative disorders, 133–137
    depersonalization/derealization disorder, 135
    dissociative amnesia, 134–135
    dissociative identity disorder (multiple personality disorder), 136–137
    other specified dissociative disorder, 137
Dissociative fugue, 134
DMDD (disruptive mood dysregulation disorder), 46–47
Donepezil (Aricept), 208
Dopamine hypothesis for schizophrenia, 26–27
Down syndrome, 121
    increases risk of developing Alzheimer disease in midlife, 104
Downward drift hypothesis, 26
Doxepin (Sinequan), 196
DPD (dependent personality disorder), 74–75
DPSD (delayed sleep phase disorder), 169
Dream interpretation, 185
Dronabinol
    FDA-approved pill form of THC, 93
Drug interactions, 192–193
Drugs of abuse
    pocket card, 7–8
DSM-5, 19
DTs (delirium tremens)
    pocket card, 9
Duloxetine (Cymbalta), 40, 195
Duty to warn, 212
Dyssomnias, 163–168
    central sleep apnea, 165–166
    circadian rhythm sleep-wake disorders, 168
    hypersomnolence disorder, 164–165
    insomnia disorder, 163–164
    narcolepsy, 167–168
    obstructive sleep apnea hypopnea, 165
    sleep-related hypoventilation, 166
Dysthymia, 44–45
Dystonia, 192

E

Eating disorders, 153–159
    anorexia nervosa, 155–157
    binge-eating disorder, 158–159
    bulimia nervosa, 157–158
    definition, 154
Ebstein's anomaly, 203
Echolalia, 25, 126
Echopraxia, 25
Effexor (venlafaxine), 40
Ego, 182
Ego-dystonic, 64
Ego-syntonic, 64, 76
Elder abuse, 118
Electroconvulsive therapy (ECT), 43, 209
Elimination disorders, 129–130
Emancipated minors
    decision making, 213

Encopresis, 129
Endocrinopathies, 23
Enuresis, 129
EPS (extrapyramidal side effects), 28, 192
Erectile disorder, 176–177
Escitalopram (Lexapro), 40
Estrogen, 174
Eszopiclone (Lunesta), 206
Examination and diagnosis, 11–20
    bedside cognitive testing, 17
        Mini-Mental State Examination (MMSE), 17
        Montreal Cognitive Assessment (MOCA), 17–18
    diagnosis and classification, 19
    diagnostic testing, 19–20
        intelligence tests, 19
        objective personality assessment tests, 19
        projective (personality) assessment tests, 20
    history, taking, 12–13
    interviewing skills, 17–19
        delusional patient, 18
        depressed patient, 19
        violent patient, 17–18
    mental status examination, 12–17
        affect, 14
        appearance/behavior, 14
        cognition, 16
        insight, 16
        interviewing, 12–13
        judgment, 16
        mood, 14
        perceptual disturbances, 15
        speech, 14
        thought content, 15
        thought process, 15
Excoriation (skin-picking) disorder, 60
Exelon (rivastigmine), 208
Exhibitionistic disorder, 179
Extrapyramidal side effects (EPS), 28, 192

F

Factitious disorder, 143–144
Family therapy, 189
    major depressive disorder, 41
    schizophrenia, 28
Fanapt (iloperidone), 28, 202
Female orgasmic disorder, 176–177
Female sexual interest/arousal disorder, 176
Fetal alcohol syndrome (FAS), 122
Fetishistic disorder, 179
First-generation (or typical) antipsychotic medications, 28
Five A's of schizophrenia, 24
Flat affect, 14, 24
Flight of ideas, 15
Flooding, 186
Flumazenil, for treating benzodiazepine overdose, 90
Fluoxetine (Prozac), 40, 194
Fluphenazine (Prolixin), 28, 199–200
Fluvoxamine (Luvox), 194
Forensic psychiatry, 211–217
    admission to a psychiatric hospital, 215
    child and family law, 217
    competence to stand trial, 215–216
    confidentiality, 212
    correctional psychiatry, 217
    decision making, 213–215
        decisional capacity, 214
        emancipated minors, 213
        guardians and conservators, 215
    disability, 215
    malingering, 217
    not guilty by reason of insanity (NGRI), 216
    risk assessment, 216–217
    standard of care and malpractice, 212
Formal neuropsychological testing, 120
Four Ds of malpractice, 212
Four Ps (predisposing to, precipitating, perpetuating, protecting), 13
Four Rs of informed consent, 213
Four-way therapy, 189
Fragile X syndrome, 121
Free association, 185
Freud, Sigmund, 182
Freud's theories of the mind, 182
Frontotemporal degeneration (FTD), 106–107
Frotteuristic disorder, 179
Fugue, 134

G

Gabapentin (Neurontin), 205
Gabitril (tiagabine), 205
Galantamine (Razadyne), 208
Gambling disorder, 95
    diagnosis and DSM-5 criteria, 95
    epidemiology/etiology, 95
    treatment, 95
Gamma-hydroxybutyrate (date-rape drug), 89
Gender dysphoria, 178
Gender identity disorder, 178
Generalized anxiety disorder (GAD), 56–57
    mnemonic: Worry WARTS, 56
Genito-pelvic pain/penetration disorder, 176, 178
Geodon (ziprasidone), 28, 202
Geriatric psychiatry, 111–118
    bereavement, 115
    dementia, 116–117
        visual hallucinations suggest Lewy body disease, 116–117
    elder abuse, 118
    major depression, 112
    medications, 118
    normal aging, 112
    nursing homes, 118
    patients with psychotic symptoms carefully evaluate for delirium, 23
    pseudodementia, 112–113
        versus dementia, 113
    restraints, 118
    sleep disturbance, 117–118
        normal sleep changes, 117
    substance use, 115–116
        alcohol and medication interactions, 116

Global developmental delay, 121
Grandeur, delusions of, 15, 22
Grief, normal, 115
Group therapy, 188–189
   in schizophrenia, 28
   sexual dysfunctions and paraphilic disorders, 177
Guanfacine
   tic disorders, 127
Guardians and conservators
   decision making, 215
Guilt, delusions of, 22

H

Hallucinations, 15, 22
Hallucinogens, 92
   intoxication, 92
   withdrawal, 92
Haloperidol (Haldol), 28, 199–200
   delirium, 101
HAM side effects, 192
HD (Huntington disease), 107–108
Heterocyclic antidepressants, 196
History, taking, 12–13
Histrionic personality disorder (HPD), 71–72
HIV infection, 107
Hoarding disorder, 59
Homicidal ideation, 15
Humor, 183
Huntington disease (HD), 107–108
Hydroxyzine (Atarax), 207
Hyperprolactinemia, 192
Hypersomnolence disorder, 164–165
Hypertensive crisis, 192, 197
Hypnagogic hallucination, 167
Hypnosis, for sexual dysfunctions and paraphilic disorders, 177
Hypokinesia, 14
Hypomanic episodes, 37, 43
Hypnopompic hallucination, 167

I

"ICU triad," 98
Id, 182
Ideas of reference, 22
Illness anxiety disorder, 142
Illusions, 15
Iloperidone (Fanapt), 28, 202
Imagery rehearsal therapy, 171
Imipramine (Tofranil), 196
Immature defenses, 184
Implosion, 186
Impulse control disorders, 147–150
   intermittent explosive disorder, 149
   kleptomania, 149–150
   overview, 148
   pyromania, 150
IMPULSIVE acronym for symptoms of borderline personality disorder, 70

Inhalants, 93
   intoxication, 93
   withdrawal, 93
Insanity, 216
Insight, 16
Insomnia disorder, 163–164
Intellectual disability, 120–121
Intellectualization, 183–184
Intelligence quotient (IQ), 19
Intelligence tests, 19
Intermittent explosive disorder, 149
Interpersonal therapy, 185
   major depressive disorder, 41
Interviewing, 17–19
   delusional patient, 18
   depressed patient, 19
   mental status examination, 12–13
   violent patient, 17–18
Intoxication
   acute intoxication and withdrawal, 80–81
   alcohol (EtOH), 82–83
   amphetamines, 88
   cocaine, 87
   hallucinogens, 92
   inhalants, 93
   marijuana, 92–93
   opioids, 90–91
   phencyclidine (PCP), 89
   sedative-hypnotics, 89–90
Invega (paliperidone), 200, 202
Involuntary admission, 215
IQ (intelligence quotient), 19
Isocarboxazid (Marplan), 197
Isolation of affect, 183
Isoniazid
   may cause psychosis, 209

J

Jet lag disorder, 169
Judgment, 16

K

Kaufman Assessment Battery for Children (K-ABC), 120
Ketamine infusion, 210
Klein, Melanie, 182
Kleptomania, 149–150
   patients frequently also suffer from bulimia nervosa, 150
Klonopin (Clonazepam), 206
Kohut, Heinz, 182
Koro, 32
Korsakoff's psychosis, 84
Korsakoff syndrome, 87
Kübler-Ross, Elisabeth, 115

L

La belle indifference, 141
Labile affect, 15

Lamotrigine (Lamictal), 204–105
Latuda (lurasidone), 28, 202
Learning theory, 186
Lewy body disease (LBD), 105–106
Lexapro (escitalopram), 40
Light therapy, 210
Lithium, 203
    bipolar I disorder, 43
        reduces suicide risk, 43
    side effects of, 43
    toxicity, pocket card for, 9
Loosening of associations, 15
Lorazepam (Ativan), 206
Loxapine (Loxitane), 199
LSD flashback, 92
Lunesta (eszopiclone), 206
Lurasidone (Latuda), 28, 202
Luvox (fluvoxamine), 194
Lyrica (pregabalin), 205

M

Mahler, Margaret, 182
Maintena (aripiprazole), 28, 200, 202
Major depressive disorder (MDD), 39–41
    course and prognosis, 40
    diagnosis and DSM-5 criteria, 39
    epidemiology, 39
    etiology, 39–40
    geriatric patients, 112
    pocket card, 7
    sleep problems associated with, 39
    treatment, 40–41
        electroconvulsive therapy (ECT), 41
        hospitalization, 40
        pharmacotherapy, 40–41
        psychotherapy, 41
Major depressive episode (MDE), 36
Maladaptive, 64
Male hypoactive sexual desire disorder, 176
Malingering, 144–145, 217
Malpractice, 212
Mania, pocket card for, 7
Manic-depression, 42
Manic episode, 36–37, 42
MAOIs (monoamine oxidase inhibitors), 40, 197–198
    major depressive disorders, 41
Marijuana, 92–93
    intoxication, 92–93
    withdrawal, 93
Marplan (isocarboxazid), 197
Mature defenses, 183
MDD (major depressive disorder). *See* Major depressive disorder (MDD)
MDE (major depressive episode), 36
Mechanical therapies, for sexual dysfunctions, 177–178
Medications. *See* Psychopharmacology
Melancholic features, 41, 44
Mellaril (thioridazine), 199
Memantine (Namenda), 208
Mental disability, 215

Mental impairment, 215
Mental status examination, 12–17
    affect, 14
    appearance/behavior, 14
    cognition, 16
    insight, 16
    interviewing, 12–13
    judgment, 16
    mood, 14
    perceptual disturbances, 15
    pocket card for, 5
    speech, 14
    thought content, 15
    thought process, 15
Methadone, for opioid use disorder, 91
"Meth mouth" (tooth decay from chronic amphetamine use), 88
Methylphenidate (Ritalin, Concerta), 207
Midazolam (Versed), 206
Mini-Mental State Examination (MMSE), 17
    pocket card, 6
Mini Mental State Exam (MMSE), 102
Minnesota Multiphasic Personality Inventory (MMPI-2), 19
Mirtazapine (Remeron), 40
    good for treating major depression in the elderly, 196
Modafinil (Provigil), 207
Molindone (Modan), 199
Monoamine oxidase inhibitors (MAOIs), 40, 197–198
    major depressive disorders, 41
Montreal Cognitive Assessment (MOCA), 17–18
Mood, 14, 36
    mental status examination, 14
Mood congruent, 36
Mood disorders, 35–47
    bereavement, 42
    bipolar I disorder, 42–43
    bipolar II disorder, 43–44
    cyclothymic disorder, 45–46
    disruptive mood dysregulation disorder (DMDD), 46–47
    due to other medical conditions, 37–38
    major depressive disorder (MDD), 39–41
    mood episodes, 36–37
        differences between manic and hypomanic episodes, 37
        hypomanic episode, 37
        major depressive episode (MDE), 36
        manic episode, 36–37
        mixed features, 37
    overview, 36
    persistent depressive disorder (dysthymia), 44–45
    premenstrual dysphoric disorder, 46
    specifiers
        bipolar disorders, 44
        depressive disorders, 41–42
    substance/medication-induced, 38
Mood stabilizers, 203
    lithium, 203
Motility, 14
Münchhausen syndrome, 144

Münchhausen syndrome by proxy, 144
Myoclonus, 109

N

Naloxone, 82, 91
Naltrexone
    opioid use disorder, 91–92
Namenda (memantine), 208
Narcissistic personality disorder
    (NPD), 72–73
Narcolepsy, 167–168
Nardil (phenelzine), 197
Navane (thiothixene), 199
Needle sharing, 90
Nefazodone (Serzone), 195
Negative reinforcement, 186
Negative symptoms of schizophrenia, 24
    Five A's, 24
Neglect, 131
Negligence, 212
Neologisms, 15, 27
Neurocognitive disorders, 97–110
    definition, 98
    delirium, 98–100
        clinical manifestations, 99
        diagnosis, 100
        epidemiology, 98
        etiology, 98
        precipitating factors, 98
        risk factors, 98
        treatment, 100–101
    mild and major neurocognitive
        disorders, 101–110
        Alzheimer disease (AD), 103–104
        clinical scenarios, 103
        diagnosis, 102–103
        DSM-5 criteria, 102
        frontotemporal degeneration (FTD), 106–107
        HIV infection, 107
        Huntington disease (HD), 107–108
        Lewy body disease (LBD), 105–106
        normal pressure hydrocephalus
            (NPH), 109–110
        Parkinson disease (PD), 108–109
        prion disease, 109
        vascular disease (vascular cognitive
            impairment), 104–105
Neuroleptic malignant syndrome
    (NMS), 29, 106, 192, 201
    pocket card, 9
Neurontin (gabapentin), 205
Neurotic defenses, 183–184
NGRI (not guilty by reason of insanity), 216
Nicotine, 94–95
    treatment of nicotine dependence, 94–95
Nifedipine
    may cause depression, 209
Nightmare disorder, 170–171
Non-BDZ anxiolytics, 207
Non-BDZ hypnotics, 206–207
Non-REM sleep arousal disorders, 169

Normal pressure hydrocephalus (NPH), 109–110
    clinical manifestations, 110
Norpramin (desipramine), 196
Nortriptyline (Pamelor, Aventyl), 196
Not guilty by reason of insanity (NGRI), 216
Nursing homes, 118
Nutritional/vitamin deficiency states, 23
Nystagmus, 89

O

OBEDIENT acronym for symptoms of dependent personality
    disorder, 74
Objective personality assessment tests, 19
Obsessions, 15, 57
    common patterns, 57
Obsessive-compulsive and related disorders
    body dysmorphic disorder, 58
    excoriation (skin-picking) disorder, 60
    hoarding disorder, 59
    obsessive-compulsive disorder (OCD), 57–58
    trichotillomania (hair-pulling disorder), 59–60
Obsessive-compulsive personality disorder (OCPD), 75–76
    compared to obsessive-compulsive disorder (OCD), 58
Obstructive sleep apnea hypopnea, 165
ODD (oppositional defiant disorder), 127–128
Olanzapine (Zyprexa), 28, 202
Olfactory hallucinations, 22
On Death and Dying, 115
Operant conditioning, 186
Opioids, 90–92
    dextromethorphan (an opioid) common in cough syrup, 90
    intoxication, 90–91
    opiate use disorder, 91
    withdrawal, 91–92
Oppositional defiant disorder (ODD), 127–128
Orap (pimozide), 199
Other specified personality disorder, 76
Oxazepam (Serax), 206
Oxcarbazepine (Trileptal), 205

P

Paliperidone (Invega), 200, 202
Pamelor (nortriptyline), 196
Pancreatic cancer, depression common in patients with, 38
Panic attacks, 51–52
    smoking is a risk factor, 53
    symptoms (Da PANICS) acronym, 51
Panic disorder, 52–53
Paranoid delusions, 15, 22
Paranoid personality disorder (PPD), 65
Paraphilias, 178–179
Parasomnias, 168–172
    nightmare disorder, 170–171
    non-REM sleep arousal disorders, 169
    overview, 168–169
    REM sleep behavior disorder, 171
    restless legs syndrome, 172
    sleep terrors, 170
    sleepwalking, 169–170
    substance/medication-induced sleep disorder, 172

Parens patriae, 215
Parkinson disease (PD), 108–109
    symptoms exacerbated by antipsychotic medications, 109
Parkinsonism, 192
Paroxetine (Paxil), 194
PCP (phencyclidine), 88–89
    intoxication, 89
    withdrawal, 89
Pedophilic disorder, 179
Perceptual disturbances, 15
Performance anxiety, 51
Perphenazine (Trilafon), 28, 199
Persecution/paranoid delusions, 22
Persistent (chronic) motor or vocal tic disorder, 127
Persistent depressive disorder (dysthymia), 44–45
Personality change due to another medical condition, 76
Personality disorders, 63–77
    CAPRI mnemonic, 64
    cluster A, 65–68
        paranoid personality disorder (PPD), 65
        schizoid personality disorder, 66–67
        schizotypal personality disorder, 67–68
    cluster B, 68–73
        antisocial personality disorder, 69–70
        borderline personality disorder (BPD), 70–71
        histrionic personality disorder (HPD), 71–72
        narcissistic personality disorder (NPD), 72–73
    cluster C, 73–76
        avoidant personality disorder, 73–74
        dependent personality disorder (DPD), 74–75
        obsessive-compulsive personality disorder (OCPD), 75–76
        other specified personality disorder, 76
        personality change due to another medical condition, 76
        unspecified personality disorder, 76
    clusters, etiology and treatment of, 64–65
    definition, 64
    diagnosis and DSM-5 criteria, 64
Phencyclidine (PCP), 88–89
    intoxication, 89
    withdrawal, 89
Phenelzine (Nardil), 197
Phobias, 15
Physical abuse, 130
Pimozide (Orap), 199
Play therapy, 120
Police power, 215
Positive reinforcement, 186
Positive symptoms of schizophrenia, 24
Postpartum mania, 44
Posttraumatic stress disorder (PTSD) and acute stress disorder, 61–62
    compared, 61
    TRAUMA acronym for etiology of PTSD, 62
PPD (paranoid personality disorder), 65
Prader–Willi syndrome, 121
Prazosin, to stop nightmares, 61
Pregabalin (Lyrica), 205
Premature (early) ejaculation, 176–177
Premenstrual dysphoric disorder, 46
Pressured speech, 14, 37
Prion disease, 109
Pristiq (desvenlafaxine), 195

Problem-solving therapy
    major depressive disorder, 41
Procainamide
    may cause confusion, delirium, 209
Prodromal phase of schizophrenia, 24
Progesterone, 175
Projection, 184
Projective (personality) assessment tests, 20
Prolixin (fluphenazine), 28, 199–200
Propranolol, 207
Proverb interpretation strategy, 16
Provigil (modafinil), 207
Provisional tic disorder, 127
Prozac (fluoxetine), 40
Pseudodementia, 112–113
Psychiatric emergencies
    pocket card, 9
Psychiatric examination of children, 120
    methods of gathering information, 120
    safety assessment, 120
    sources of information, 120
Psychiatric manifestations of major neurocognitive disorders (dementia), 116–117
Psychiatric symptoms caused by particular medications, 208–209
Psychiatry, why spend time on it?, 2
Psychoanalysis, 184–185
Psychoanalytically oriented psychotherapy, 185
Psychodynamic psychotherapy
    anxiety disorders, 51
    major depressive disorder, 41
Psychoeducation
    elimination disorders, 129
Psychological abuse, 130
Psychomotor retardation, 14
Psychopharmacology, 191–210
    anticonvulsants, 204
        carbamazepine (Tegretol), 204
        valproic acid (Depakote and Depakene), 204–205
    antidepressants, 193–198
        heterocyclic antidepressants, 196
        miscellaneous antidepressants, 195–196
        monoamine oxidase inhibitors, 197–198
        selective serotonin reuptake inhibitors, 193–195
        serotonin-norepinephrine reuptake inhibitors (SNRIs), 195
        tetracyclic antidepressants, 196–197
        tricyclic antidepressants, 196
        use in other disorders, 198
    antipsychotics, 198–203
        atypical (second-generation) antipsychotics, 201–202
        typical (first-generation) antipsychotics, 199–201
    anxiolytics/hypnotics, 205–207
        benzodiazepines, 205–206
        non-BDZ anxiolytics, 207
        non-BDZ hypnotics, 206–207
    cognitive enhancers, 208
        acetylcholinesterase inhibitors, 208
        NMDA (glutamate) receptor antagonist, 208
    mood stabilizers, 203
        lithium, 203
    other treatments, 209–210
        deep brain stimulation (DBS), 209
        electroconvulsive therapy (ECT), 209

Psychopharmacology (*Continued*)
    ketamine infusion, 210
    light therapy, 210
    repetitive transcranial magnetic stimulation (rTMS), 209–210
    psychiatric symptoms caused by particular medications, 208–209
        agitation/confusion/delirium, 208
        anxiety, 208
        depression, 208
        psychosis, 208
        sedation/poor concentration, 209
    psychostimulants, 207
    side effects, 191–192
Psychosis, 22–23
    definition of, 22
    delusions, 22
    differential diagnosis, 22–23
    perceptual disturbances, 22
    psychotic disorder due to another medical condition, 23
    substance/medication-induced psychotic disorder, 23, 208
Psychostimulants, 207
Psychotherapies, 181–189
    behavioral therapy, 186
        conditioning, 186
        deconditioning, 186–187
        learning theory, 186
    cognitive-behavioral therapy (CBT), 187
        anxiety disorders, 51
        chronic insomnia, 163
        major depressive disorder, 41
        sexual dysfunctions and paraphilic disorders, 177
    couples therapy, 189
    defense mechanisms, 182–184
        immature defenses, 184
        mature defenses, 183
        neurotic defenses, 183–184
    dialectical behavior therapy (DBT), 188
    family therapy, 189
    Freud's theories of the mind, 182
    group therapy, 188–189
    overview, 182
    psychoanalysis, 184–185
Psychotic disorders, 21–33
    brief psychotic disorder, 30
    comparing
        distinguishing features, 32
        prognosis, 32
        time course, 32
    culture-specific psychoses, 32
    delusional disorder, 31
    psychosis, 22–23
        delusions, 22
        differential diagnosis, 22–23
        perceptual disturbances, 22
        psychotic disorder due to another medical condition, 23
        substance/medication-induced psychotic disorder, 23
    schizoaffective disorder, 30
    schizophrenia, 23–29
        cognitive symptoms, 24
        diagnosis, 24–25
        downward drift, 26
        epidemiology, 26
        negative symptoms, 24
        pathophysiology of schizophrenia: dopamine hypothesis, 26–27
        pathophysiology of schizophrenia: other neurotransmitter abnormalities, 27
        positive symptoms, 24
        prodromal phase, 24
        prognostic factors, 27–28
        psychiatric exam, 26
        psychotic phase, 24
        residual phase, 24
        treatment, 28–29
    schizophreniform disorder, 29–30
Psychotic features, 44
PTSD (posttraumatic stress disorder) and acute stress disorder. *See* Posttraumatic stress disorder (PTSD) and acute stress disorder
Punitive damages, 212
Pyromania, 150

Q

Quetiapine (Seroquel), 28, 202
Quirks, 64

R

Ramelteon (Rozerem), 207
Rapid cycling, 44
Rapid eye movement (REM). *See* REM (rapid eye movement)
Rationalization, 184
Razadyne (galantamine), 208
Reaction formation, 184
Recurrent major depressive episodes with hypomania, 43
RED DANES acronym for PCP intoxication symptoms, 89
Reference, ideas of, 22
Reference delusions, 15
Refractory depression, 197
Regression, 72, 75, 184
Religious delusions, 15
Remeron (mirtazapine), 40
    good for treating major depression in the elderly, 196
REM (rapid eye movement)
    sleep, 163
    sleep behavior disorder, 171
        Lewy body disease and, 105
Repetitive transcranial magnetic stimulation (rTMS), 209–210
Repression, 184
Residual phase of schizophrenia, 24
Restless legs syndrome, 172
Restoril (temazepam), 206
Restraints
    elderly patients, 118
Risk assessment, 216–217
Risperidone (Consta), 28, 200
Risperidone (Risperdal), 202
Ritalin (methylphenidate), 207
Rivastigmine (Exelon), 208

Rorschach Test, 20
Rozerem (ramelteon), 207
rTMS (repetitive transcranial magnetic stimulation), 209–210

S
SAD PERSONS (suicide risk)
    pocket card, 7
Schizoaffective disorder, 30
    distinguishing features and prognosis, 32
Schizoid disorder
    distinguishing features, 32
Schizoid personality disorder, 66–67
Schizophrenia, 23–29
    cognitive symptoms, 24
    versus delusional disorder, 31
    diagnosis, 24–25
    downward drift, 26
    epidemiology, 26
    lasts for longer than 6 months, 26
    negative symptoms, 24
    overview, 24
    pathophysiology
        dopamine hypothesis, 26–27
        other neurotransmitter abnormalities, 27
    positive symptoms, 24
    prodromal phase, 24
    prognostic factors, 27–28
    psychiatric exam, 26
    psychotic phase, 24
    residual phase, 24
    time course and prognosis, 32
    treatment, 28–29
        behavioral therapy, 28
        pharmacologic treatment, 28–29
Schizophreniform disorder, 26, 29–30
    time course and prognosis, 32
Schizotypal disorder (personality disorder), 32, 67–68
Seasonal affective disorder, 42
Seasonal pattern, 44
Secondary amines, 196
Second-generation (or atypical) antipsychotic medications, 28
Sedation/poor concentration, medications causing, 209
Sedative-hypnotics, 89–90
    intoxication, 89–90
    withdrawal, 90
Selective mutism, 54–55
Selective serotonin reuptake inhibitors (SSRIs), 40, 193–195
    anxiety disorders, 51
    binge-eating disorder, 159
    not to be used within 2 weeks before or after use of an MAOI, 51
    suicidal FDA warning, 193
Senile plaques, 104
Separation anxiety disorder, 55
Saphris (asenapine), 28
Serax (oxazepam), 206
Seroquel (quetiapine), 28, 202
Serotonin-norepinephrine reuptake inhibitors (SNRIs), 40, 195
    anxiety disorders, 51

Serotonin syndrome, 41, 90, 192, 197, 294–295
    pocket card, 9
Sertraline (Zoloft), 40, 194
Serzone (nefazodone), 195
Sex therapy, 176–177
Sexual abuse, 130
Sexual dysfunctions and paraphilic disorders, 173–179
    differential diagnosis, 174–176
    gender dysphoria, 178
    paraphilias, 178–179
    sexual changes with aging, 174
    sexual response cycle, 174
    treatment
        analytically oriented (psychodynamic) psychotherapy, 177
        cognitive-behavioral therapy, 177
        group therapy, 177
        hypnosis, 177
        mechanical therapies, 177–178
        pharmacologic treatment, 177
        sex therapy, 176–177
Sexual masochism disorder, 179
Sexual response cycle, 174
Sexual sadism disorder, 179
Shift-work disorder (SWD), 169
Side effects of medications, 191–192
SIG E. CAPS (major depression), 36
    pocket card, 7
Sinequan (doxepin), 196
Skinner, B.F., 186
Sleep-wake cycle, normal, 162
Sleep-wake disorders, 161–172
    dyssomnias, 163–168
        central sleep apnea, 165–166
        circadian rhythm sleep-wake disorders, 168
        hypersomnolence disorder, 164–165
        insomnia disorder, 163–164
        narcolepsy, 167–168
        obstructive sleep apnea hypopnea, 165
        sleep-related hypoventilation, 166
    geriatric psychiatry, 117–118
    parasomnias, 168–172
        nightmare disorder, 170–171
        non-REM sleep arousal disorders, 169
        overview, 168–169
        REM sleep behavior disorder, 171
        restless legs syndrome, 172
        sleep terrors, 170
        sleepwalking, 169–170
        substance/medication-induced sleep disorder, 172
    sleep disorders, 162
SNRIs (serotonin-norepinephrine reuptake inhibitors), 40, 195
    anxiety disorders, 51
Social anxiety disorders (social phobia), 54
SOD (social and/or occupational dysfunction), 50
Somatic delusions, 15, 22
Somatic symptom and factitious disorders, 139–145
    conversion disorder (functional neurological symptom disorder), 141–142
    factitious disorder, 143–144
    illness anxiety disorder, 142
    malingering, 144–145
    overview, 140

Somatic symptom and factitious disorders (*Continued*)
    psychological factors affecting other medical conditions, 143
    review of distinguishing features, 145
    somatic symptom disorder, 141
Sonata (Zaleplon), 206
Specific learning disorder (LD), 122
Specific phobias, 53–54
Speech, 14
Splitting, 71, 184
SSRIs (selective serotonin reuptake inhibitors). *See* Selective serotonin reuptake inhibitors (SSRIs)
Standard of care, 212
Stelazine (trifluoperazine), 199
Steroids
    significant side effects, 209
Stevens–Johnson syndrome, 204
Strattera (atomoxetine), 207
Stroke patients, at risk for developing depression, 38
Sublimation, 183
Substance/medication-induced mood disorders, 38
Substance/medication-induced sleep disorder, 172
Substance-related and addictive disorders, 79–95
    alcohol (EtOH), 82–87
        alcohol use disorder, 85–87
        clinical presentation of alcohol intoxication, 82
        intoxication, 82–83
        withdrawal, 83–84
    amphetamines, 88
        intoxication, 88
    caffeine, 94
        overdose, 94
        withdrawal, 94
    cocaine, 87–88
        cocaine use disorder, 87
        intoxication, 87
        withdrawal, 88
    gambling disorder, 95
        diagnosis and DSM-5 criteria, 95
        epidemiology/etiology, 95
        treatment, 95
    geriatric psychiatry, 115–116
    hallucinogens, 92
        intoxication, 92
        withdrawal, 92
    inhalants, 93
        intoxication, 93
        withdrawal, 93
    marijuana, 92–93
        intoxication, 92–93
        withdrawal, 93
    nicotine, 94–95
        treatment of nicotine dependence, 94–95
    opioids, 90–92
        intoxication, 90–91
        opiate use disorder, 91
        withdrawal, 91–92
    phencyclidine (PCP), 88–89
        intoxication, 89
        withdrawal, 89
    sedative-hypnotics, 89–90
        intoxication, 89–90
        withdrawal, 90
    substance use disorders, 80–81
        acute intoxication and withdrawal, 80–81
        detection, 81
        diagnosis and DSM-5 criteria, 80
        epidemiology, 80
        psychiatric symptoms, 80
        treatment, 81
Suicidal ideation, 15
Suicidality, assessing, 19
    pocket card, 7
Superego, 182
Supportive psychotherapy, 41, 185
Suppression, 183
Suprachiasmic nucleus, 168
SWD (shift-work disorder), 169
Sympathomimetics
    may cause anxiety, 208
    may cause psychosis, 209
Systematic desensitization, 186

T

Tactile delusions, 22
Tangentiality, 15
Tarasoff duty, 212
Tardive dyskinesia (TD), 28–29, 192, 201
TCAs (tricyclic antidepressants), 40, 196
    toxicity, pocket card, 9
Tegretol (carbamazepine), 204
Temazepam (Restoril), 206
Tertiary amines, 196
Testosterone, 175
Tetracyclic antidepressants, 196–197
Tetracycline
    may cause depression, 209
Thematic Apperception Test (TAT), 20
Therapeutic alliance, 185
Thioridazine (Mellaril), 199
Thiothixene (Navane), 199
Thorazine (chlorpromazine), 28, 199
Thought blocking, 15
Thought broadcasting, 15, 22
Thought content, 15
Thought insertion, 22
Thought process, 15
Three Ws of normal pressure hydrocephalus, 110
Thyroid dysfunction
    cause of reversible cognitive impairment, 102
Tiagabine (Gabitril), 205
Tic disorders, 126–127
    Tourette's disorder, 126–127
Tofranil (imipramine), 196
Token economy, 186
Tooth decay from chronic amphetamine use ("meth mouth"), 88
Topiramate (Topamax), 205
TORCH acronym for infections and toxins, 121
Tourette's disorder, 126–127
Transference, 185
Transgender, 178
Transsexuality, 178
Transvestic disorder, 179
Tranylcypromine (Parnate), 197

Trauma and stressor-related disorders, 60–62
   adjustment disorders, 62
   posttraumatic stress disorder (PTSD) and acute stress disorder, 61–62
Trazodone (Desyrel), 195–196
   causes priapism, 195–196
Triangles, 189
Trichotillomania (hair-pulling disorder), 59–60
Tricyclic antidepressants (TCAs), 40, 196
   toxicity, pocket card, 9
Trifluoperazine (Stelazine), 199
Trilafon (perphenazine), 28, 199
Trileptal (oxcarbazepine), 205
Typical (first-generation) antipsychotics, 199–201
Tyramine reaction/hypertensive crisis
   pocket card, 9

U

"Uncontrollable urges," triad of, 57
Undoing, 184
Unspecified personality disorder, 76

V

VALEUMS acronym for substance/medication intoxication, 100
Valium (diazepam), 206
Valproic acid (Depakote, Depakene), 204–205
Vascular disease (vascular cognitive impairment), 104–105
Venlafaxine (Effexor), 40, 195
Versed (midazolam), 206
Violence, 217
   prior history is most important predictor, 18
Violent patients, interviewing, 17–18
Visual hallucinations, 22
Vocabulary strategy, 16
Voluntary admission, 215
Voyeuristic disorder, 179

W

WAIS (Wechsler Adult Intelligence Scale), 19
Wards, behavior on, 2–4
   be a team player, 3
   keep patient information handy, 3
   present patient information in an organized manner, 3–4
   respect patients' rights, 3
   respect the field of psychiatry, 2
   respect the patients, 2
   take responsibility for your patients, 2–3
   volunteer, 3
Warn, duty to, 212
Wechsler Adult Intelligence Scale (WAIS), 19
Wechsler Intelligence Scale for Children (WISC), 19
Wechsler Intelligence Scale for Children-Revised (WISC-R), 120
Wernicke's encephalopathy, 87
Withdrawal
   alcohol (EtOH), 83–84
   caffeine, 94
   cocaine, 88
   hallucinogens, 92
   inhalants, 93
   marijuana, 93
   opioids, 91–92
   phencyclidine (PCP), 89
   sedative-hypnotics, 90
Word salad, 15

X

Xanax (alprazolam), 206

Z

Zaleplon (Sonata), 206
Ziprasidone (Geodon), 28, 202
Zoloft (sertraline), 40
Zolpidem (Ambien), 206
Zyprexa (olanzapine), 28, 202